PUBLIC HEALTH IN THE 21ST CENTURY

ADOLESCENT HEALTH LITERACY AND LEARNING

PUBLIC HEALTH IN THE 21ST CENTURY

Additional books in this series can be found on Nova's website
under the Series tab.

Additional e-books in this series can be found on Nova's website
under the e-book tab.

PUBLIC HEALTH IN THE 21ST CENTURY

ADOLESCENT HEALTH LITERACY AND LEARNING

DEBORAH L. BEGORAY
AND
ELIZABETH M. BANISTER
EDITORS

nova publishers
New York

Library of Congress Cataloging-in-Publication Data

ISBN: 978-1-63482-897-0
Library of Congress Control Number: 2015939635

Published by Nova Science Publishers, Inc. † New York

To the memory of Edward John Wigmore, much-loved uncle, mentor, and friend

— Deborah

CONTENTS

FOREWORD: HEALTH LITERACY IN ADOLESCENT CONTEXTS

*Irving Rootman**

Adjunct Professor in the School of Public Health and Social Policy,
University of Victoria, and a Visiting Professor in the Department of Gerontology,
Simon Fraser University, Canada

The field of health literacy has advanced considerably over the past decade. Among other things, there has been a growing consensus among people working in the field that health literacy cannot be understood without taking context into account. In part, this was stimulated by the U.S. Institute of Medicine Expert Committee on Health Literacy report (2004) that, among other things, suggested "Health literacy emerges when the expectations, preferences, and skills of individuals seeking health information and services meet the expectations, preferences and skills of those providing information and services" (p. 2). The committee also provided a framework that illustrated the "interaction of individuals with education systems, health systems, and societal factors as they relate to health literacy" and referred to them as "Health Contexts" (p. 33). Since then, researchers and practitioners in Canada and elsewhere have used the term *contexts* or sometimes *settings* to refer to this interaction.

This book builds on the idea of context to analyze the unique experiences of adolescents in Canada and other, mainly developed countries in relation to health literacy. In particular, it carefully looks at the challenges and barriers adolescents often confront as well as the social, cultural, and ecological factors that affect their abilities to access, understand, evaluate, and communicate health information that helps them to inform themselves and make decisions related to their health. The authors also consider contexts in which health, education, and other information providers obtain health information and convey it to adolescents in a manner that is both engaging and effective. In particular, they focus on some contexts that are relevant to adolescents including gender, mental health, socioeconomic status, and culture. In addition to using the idea of contexts in relation to adolescents, the book helps to advance the field of health literacy conceptually and practically.

* irootman@telus.net

From a conceptual point of view, one chapter presents a critical appraisal of definitions of adolescent health literacy and concludes that "definitions of adolescent health literacy are needed to clearly distinguish how it differs from health literacy in children and adults" (Malloy-Weir, chapter 2, p. 4). To this end, she suggests adopting "stipulative definitions" and benchmarks. Another chapter introduces the concept of "critical media health literacy" and presents a conceptual framework for research based on this kind of health literacy, which may be particularly important for adolescents — many of whom are heavy users of social media (Beer & Begoray, chapter 4, p. 12). A third chapter presents a "re-envisioned" definition of mental health literacy based on a critical literacy perspective that includes "collective knowledges, meanings and experiences of mental health that aid in awareness … and transformation … and that enable emancipatory action … and full participation … in maintaining and enhancing mental wellness across variable, localized contexts" (Ranahan, chapter 8, p. 9). Not only is this definition helpful for research in mental health literacy but, perhaps more importantly, it may contribute significantly to developing and implementing more effective ways of addressing "wild" youth issues such as suicide. Another chapter uses a conceptualization of health literacy to reveal "students' insights into accessing, understanding, evaluating, and communicating health information;" on that basis, the authors argue that "secondary curricula need to accommodate the gendered nature of youth health literacy needs" (Wharf Higgins & Bellows Riecken, chapter 6, p. 1).

The book also suggests a number of specific ways of working with adolescents on health literacy based on research evidence. For example, one chapter presents a study of the use of a graphic novel developed by a group of "middle years" students as a way to engage another group of students from a middle school in a lower socioeconomic area in a critical analysis of media advertising focusing on gender differences. The authors state that the use of the novel was both effective and engaging and that the "teacher's dialogic approach might be adopted by health care professionals as a way to engage adolescents in discussing health issues" (Begoray & Fu, chapter 3, p. 13). Another chapter presents an analysis of a hands-on creative project involving art materials to help middle school adolescents reflect critically on the interaction of gender with health advertising and reports that such an approach was "valid for pedagogy in middle years' classrooms" (Banister & Begoray, chapter 5, p. 10). A third chapter presents an analysis of eleven award-winning novels for middle and high school students and concludes that "not only are problem novels useful for adolescent girls' learning but will also help educate adults about the modern health concerns of these girls" (Begoray, Banister, & Jaswal, chapter 9, p. 1).

One chapter focuses on the role of culture in relation to mental health literacy among Aboriginal adolescents. Among other things, the author concludes that "Culturally relevant and culturally safe mental health approaches, programs, and resources can engage and empower Aboriginal youth to recognize their strengths and support them along the past of mental wellness" (Marshall, chapter 7, p. 1).

In addition, the book contains a number of educational features that make it particularly useful for students and others. These include *Focusing Questions* at the beginning of every chapter, *Discussion Questions* and a *List of Online Resources* at the end of the chapter, and suggested exercises and activities for educators and parents. As noted in the introductory chapter, this book has many insights and ideas that will be of interest to other audiences, including coaches, parents, grandparents, policymakers, and citizens in general. To this list, I would add people working in the field of health literacy who would benefit greatly by seeing an innovative, positive, comprehensive, evidence-based approach to research and practice in the field related to adolescent contexts.

Reference

Institute of Medicine Committee on Health Literacy. (2004). *Health literacy: A prescription to end confusion* (L. Nielsen-Bohlman, A. M. Panzer, & D. A. Kindig, Eds.). Washington, DC: National Academy of Sciences.

Authors' Biographical Information

Editors

Deborah L. Begoray, PhD, is a Professor of Language and Literacy in the Department of Curriculum and Instruction, Faculty of Education, University of Victoria, British Columbia, Canada. She does literacy and health literacy teaching and research in a variety of contexts and with a wide range of learners especially adolescents. She also leads interdisciplinary project teams and works with preservice and inservice teachers. Deborah is the lead recipient of both SSHRC and CIHR grants to support her research as a community engaged scholar. Deborah writes extensively on literacy research in Aboriginal and non-Aboriginal communities, both rural and urban, where she is currently looking at the use of adolescent-produced graphic novels as curricular resources and research dissemination tools. Her previous publications on health literacy include her work as lead editor of *Health Literacy in Context: International Perspectives* (2012) and lead author of *Mediating Health: The Powerful Role of the Media as Adolescent Health Literacy Educator* (2009).
dbegoray@uvic.ca
Affiliation: University of Victoria, Department of Curriculum and Instruction
Academic Title: Professor

Elizabeth M. Banister, RN, PhD, RPsych, is a Professor of Nursing in the School of Nursing, Faculty of Human and Social Development, University of Victoria, British Columbia, Canada. Her research interests include knowledge translation, adolescent sexual health literacy, media health literacy, health education, and qualitative research design. She teaches advanced practice nurses a wide range of topics including health literacy and knowledge translation. She served on the Advisory Board for the Canadian Institutes of Health Research (CIHR) Institute of Gender and Health (IGH) for six years and has multidisciplinary research collaborations in Canada and New Zealand. Her publications focus on adolescent sexual health literacy, media health literacy, and gender and health in Aboriginal and non-Aboriginal communities. She is lead editor of *Knowledge Translation in Context: Indigenous, Policy, and Community Settings* (2011).
ebaniste@uvic.ca
Affiliation: University of Victoria, School of Nursing
Academic Title: Professor

AUTHORS

Christine Beer, PhD, is a health promotion researcher and designer of disease surveillance software applications based in Victoria, British Columbia, Canada. Her main interests include the promotion of healthy adolescence, mindfulness-based stress reduction, and disease prevention. Chris researches the influences of social media and health literacy on adolescents' health performance, and she conducts stress reduction workshops for high school students and workplace groups.
beercm@gmail.com
Affiliation: IBM Global Consulting Services
Academic Title: Independent Researcher

Kai Bellows Riecken, PhD, studied psychology at the undergraduate level at the University of Victoria, British Columbia, Canada, and later moved on to graduate studies in its School of Exercise Science, Physical and Health Education (EPHE). Kai's doctoral research focused on health literacy, physical activity, school-based health initiatives, and action-based research. She has been a term instructor at the University of Victoria and Camosun College over the past six years and has worked on a variety of longitudinal health research projects. Presently, Kai is fulfilling a three-year contract conducting an evaluation for a health-promoting school initiative via several health authorities.
kaib@uvic.ca
Affiliation: University of Victoria, School of Exercise Science, Physical and Health Education
Academic Title: Independent Researcher

Hong Fu, MA, is a doctoral student in the Faculty of Education, University of Victoria, British Columbia, Canada. Hong has experience in teaching English as a foreign language in international contexts. Her research interest and experience in her doctoral study includes teacher identity, critical theory and critical pedagogy, feminist post structuralism, media literacy, teaching and learning theories, education and technology (e.g., e-portfolios). Hong performs literature review writing, interviewing and data collecting, and analysis in multiple research projects in the capacity of a research assistant.
fuhong@uvic.ca
Affiliation: University of Victoria, Department of Curriculum and Instruction
Academic Title: Doctoral Candidate

Sabrena Jaswal, MA, is a workplace health coordinator in local government in the United Kingdom. She has over ten years of experience in the field of qualitative research in the areas of health and health literacy; she has undertaken research and research evaluations in the areas of health and health literacy with young people, individuals at risk of cardiovascular disease, and health professionals in the disciplines of public health and midwifery. Sabrena's research interests include doctor-patient communication with an emphasis on examining the social rules regarding communication and how these rules

can facilitate or impede a person's health care, service user engagement, and medical school curriculum in relation to communication.
sabrenajaswal@outlook.com
Affiliation: Adur & Worthing Councils, Communities, West Sussex, England
Academic title: Independent Researcher

Leslie Malloy-Weir, MA, is a PhD Candidate in the Health Policy program, Department of Clinical Epidemiology & Biostatistics, McMaster University, Hamilton, Ontario, Canada. For her master's research, she examined predictors of health literacy in older adults and the role of health literacy in Internet searches for health information, using data from the 2003 Canadian version of the International Adult Literacy and Life Skills Survey. For her doctoral research, she identified 250 different definitions of health literacy in the academic literature. Leslie also examined empirical relationships between health literacy and numeracy and the three stages of the treatment decision-making process. In 2015, Leslie completed a Science Policy Fellowship at Health Canada.
malloylj@mcmaster.ca
Affiliation: McMaster University, Department of Clinical Epidemiology & Biostatistics
Academic Title: Doctoral Candidate

E. Anne Marshall, PhD, RPsych, is a Professor of Counselling Psychology in the Department Educational Psychology and Leadership Studies and the Provost's Community Engaged Scholar at the University of Victoria, British Columbia, Canada. She is also Director of the University's Centre for Youth & Society, an interdisciplinary research centre that is dedicated to improving the lives of youth and families in diverse societal circumstances. Anne is the co-developer of the Indigenous Communities Counselling Psychology graduate program, the first of its kind in Canada. Her own community-engaged research projects focus on youth mental health in cultural contexts, educational and work transitions, and qualitative methods. Much of her work involves Indigenous communities and marginalized youth populations. Anne is co-editor of *Knowledge Translation in Context: Indigenous, Policy, and Community Settings* (2011).
amarshal@uvic.ca
Affiliation: University of Victoria, Department of Educational Psychology and Leadership Studies
Academic Title: Professor

Patti Ranahan, PhD, is an Assistant Professor in the Department of Applied Human Sciences, Concordia University, Montreal, Québec, Canada. Her research examines mental health literacy for youth work practice, youth work pedagogical approaches, and attachment-based interventions with francophone parents to address adolescent mental health issues. Drawing from her professional experience as a youth work practitioner and informed by her research, Patti designs and instructs graduate and undergraduate courses in mental health and addictions, case management and supervision, and fundamentals of child and youth care work.
patti.ranahan@concordia.ca
Affiliation: Concordia University, Department of Applied Human Sciences
Academic Title: Assistant Professor

Irving Rootman, Ph.D., LLD (Hon.), is an Adjunct Professor in the School of Public Health and Social Policy, University of Victoria, and a Visiting Professor in the Department of Gerontology, Simon Fraser University, British Columbia, Canada. Irv has been a researcher, research manager, program manager, professor, and consultant in the field of health promotion for more than 30 years. Currently, he is the co-chair of the Capacity-building Committee for the Public Health Association of British Columbia as well as the chair of the Steering Committee for the BC Health Literacy Network. Irv was a member of the U.S. Institute of Medicine Expert Committee on Health Literacy and co-chair of the Canadian Expert Panel on Health Literacy. He has conducted research on health literacy and published numerous papers and articles on the topic since 2003.

irootman@telus.net

Affiliations: University of Victoria, School of Public Health and Social Policy; Simon Fraser University, Department of Gerontology

Academic Title: Adjunct Professor; Visiting Professor, respectively

Joan Wharf Higgins, PhD, is a Professor in the School of Exercise Science, Physical and Health Education, University of Victoria, British Columbia, Canada, where she held a Canada Research Chair from 2004–2014. Her areas of research include health literacy, social marketing, healthy living, and health promotion/chronic disease prevention. Joan prefers carrying out 'real world research' conducted in, for, and with communities. In her leisure time, Joan is a long-distance runner.

jwharfhi@uvic.ca

Affiliation: University of Victoria, School of Exercise Science, Physical and Health Education

Academic Title: Professor

In: Adolescent Health Literacy and Learning
Editors: D. L. Begoray and E. M. Banister ISBN: 978-1-63482-897-0

Chapter 1

WHY FOCUS ON ADOLESCENT HEALTH LITERACY AND LEARNING?

***Deborah Begoray*[*1] *and Elizabeth Banister*[2]**
[1]Department of Curriculum and Instruction, University of Victoria, Canada
[2]School of Nursing, University of Victoria, Canada

ABSTRACT

The purpose of this chapter is to give background for reading the chapters that follow in this book. To that end, we begin with a discussion of adolescence, adolescent health, and adolescent health literacy. We then consider how adolescents learn and how, therefore, they might achieve greater health literacy with the facilitation of skilled instructors in schools, clinics, and in other health-related contexts. Health education is a matter certainly for the formal education system and the government, which mandates curricula, but also for parents and for health practitioners in the wider community.

Keywords: adolescents, health literacy, learning, health education

INTRODUCTION

Focusing Questions

1. Why do you think adolescent health literacy is important?
2. How do you think adolescents might best be engaged in learning about health literacy and becoming more health literate?

This book is being written at a time when adolescent health is at a crucial juncture. The health of adolescents is of increasing concern around the world (World Health Organization [WHO], 2014). Behaviours that concern nutrition, sex, substance misuse, exercise, and

[*] Correspondence to (email): dbegoray@uvic.ca.

chronic illness self-management that are adopted during adolescence (Viner et al., 2012) can have long-term consequences in future life stages.

There is, however, a scarcity of research on adolescent health literacy and a lack of inquiries on what interventions might be useful in educational contexts (Manganello, 2008; Perry, 2014) to improve health literacy in adolescents. Clearly then, we need to raise the profile of adolescent health literacy and learning if we are to begin to address issues in adolescent health. Mental health challenges are common in adolescents of all economic backgrounds; far too often, their particular needs are not being met (Marcus & Westra, 2012). Gender influences are also significant: adolescent boys and girls encounter health questions and messages differently. And while we try in our schools and clinics to help adolescents to become more health-literate, the commercial media is a powerful health educator (Begoray, Cimon, & Wharf Higgins, 2010) whose messages are aggressive, ubiquitous, and often encourage risky health behaviours.

What Is Adolescence?

Adolescence, a term much debated, is defined by the WHO as the period between childhood and adulthood from 10 to 19 years old and characterized by major biological, psychological, and social changes (Gray, Culpepper, & Welsh, 2012). It is characterized by multiple transitions, including biological changes, and changes in cognitive skills, emotional development, social roles, and identity (Kaufman, 2006). These transitions interact, influencing adolescent health and well-being (Viner et al., 2012) as well as an adolescent's ability to make health decisions (Suleiman & Brindis, 2014) with greater independence. In addition, we know that "[t]he critical period for the acquisition of health literacy is during adolescence, when health and biology subject matter are acquired, metacognition develops, and health and well-being behaviours are in their formative stages" (Blanton & Wood, 2009, p. 4). This is our opportunity to work with adolescents to improve their health literacy and, in turn, health outcomes.

What Health Challenges and Barriers Confront Adolescents?

Adolescents confront a variety of health problems. Worldwide, more than 2 million adolescents are living with HIV and approximately 1.3 million adolescents died in 2012 from causes that could be prevented or treated (WHO, 2014). Motor vehicle injuries to adolescents were the leading cause of death amongst non-Aboriginal adolescents — amongst whom it was the second leading cause — in 2012 with approximately 330 deaths every day. Other main causes of death are HIV, suicide, lower respiratory infections, and interpersonal violence (WHO, 2014). Mental health problems are widespread in North American children and adolescents (Canadian Mental Health Association, 2014; National Institute of Mental Health, n.d.); the problem is especially acute worldwide in Aboriginal young adult populations (Price & Dalgleish, 2013), where suicide is the leading cause of death. In the United States, adolescent pregnancy rates continue to be one of the highest in the developed world; for example, they are twice as high as rates in Canada and Sweden (Guttmacher Institute, 2014). Alcohol and substance abuse is yet another risk that is disproportionately high for adolescents. According to Health Canada (2012), "[o]ne in four (24.4%) youth drinkers versus 17.6% of adult drinkers exceeded the guideline for chronic risk, while the acute-risk guideline was exceeded by 17.9% of youth drinkers and 11.9% of adult drinkers." (§ Low-risk alcohol use, para. 3) and "[t]he prevalence of reported harm due to their own drug use was four times higher among youth aged 15 to 24 years (5.5%) than adults aged 25 years and older (1.4%)." (§ Harms related to illicit drug use, para. 1). Chronic diseases such as diabetes that at one time began in mid to late adulthood are becoming more prevalent in younger ages (Van Cleave, Gortmaker, & Perrin, 2010; Zimmet, 2011).

Structural factors (e.g., income and access to education) have a significant influence on the health of adolescents (Lê, Roux, & Morgenstern, 2012). There are approximately two billion adolescents globally of whom 86% live in low-income and middle-income countries (United Nations Fund for Population Activities, 2011) and millions of these have no access to formal education. Low education levels are associated with poor health (Viner et al., 2012) — even in relatively wealthy countries such as Canada and the United States.

WHAT IS ADOLESCENT HEALTH LITERACY?

Rootman and Gordon-El-Bihbety (2008) offered the general definition that health literacy is the ability "to access, understand, evaluate, and communicate information as a way to promote, maintain, and improve health in a variety of settings across the life-course" (p. 3). Health literacy allows individuals to make informed decisions about their health (Matthews, Kilgour, Christian, Mori, & Hill, 2014) based on skills needed to acquire and maintain good health (Nutbeam, 2000). Adolescence is, of course, part of the life-course with its own particular challenges, depending on such additional variables as gender, socioeconomic status, and cultural background. Adolescent health literacy is influenced by a social ecology (Wharf Higgins, Begoray, & MacDonald, 2009) of family and friends, teachers and coaches. Adolescent health literacy education is a concern for community health care professionals such as school nurses (Smart, Parker, Lampert, & Sulo, 2012), clinic nurses (Banister, Begoray, & Daly, 2011), and pediatricians (Rothman et al., 2009) as well as for government policies and the global media. In adolescence, teens are setting the attitudes and behaviours about their health that persist into adulthood (Kolbe, 2005).

HOW DO ADOLESCENTS LEARN AND WHAT ARE THE IMPLICATIONS FOR HEALTH EDUCATORS?

Health literacy is one of the 21st century interdisciplinary themes for learning promoted by the Partnership for 21st Century Skills (2011). Health education plays an important role in enhancing individuals' health literacy (WHO, 2012). Adolescents need access to health education in order to make healthy choices in life and to take an active role in the community (Persson & Haraldsson, 2013). By influencing their abilities and offering support, "meaningful and sustained change" in their health can take place (WHO, 2012, p. 6) throughout their lifespan. Adolescents need to have good health in order to learn and function as effective citizens of the community and of society (Persson & Haraldsson, 2013).

Learning contexts and themes that promote a sense of belonging (Anderman, 2002), are socially engaging, and promote positive interactions with peers influence learning outcomes for adolescents. Adolescents are more likely to learn when they are working in cooperative groups with peers, have flexibility with choice of learning content (Anderman, Sinatra, & Gray, 2012), and experience positive interactions with teachers (Reeve, 2009; Smart et al., 2012). Adolescent learning is enhanced in learning situations that encourage inquiry-based learning (Chinn & Malhotra, 2002; Paakkari & Paakkari, 2012) focused on areas of personal relevance. Inquiry projects that allow the use of technology for searching out health information and communicating with others about health are of particular interest to 21st century adolescents (Suleiman & Brindis, 2014). Health education, therefore, needs to feature a "greater understanding of [adolescents'] aspirations and concerns" (Blum, Bastos, Kabiru, & Le, 2012, p. 379) and preferred approaches to learning than it does currently. Improving adolescent health literacy and learning has important roles for both adult experts and adolescents themselves.

Health education has a positive influence on health literacy and in health outcomes for adolescents. Health education in schools, however, is often minimal. For example, in British Columbia (BC), Canada, high school students only have a recommended 36 hours of health education (BC Ministry of Education, 2007). Research suggests that health literacy-based curricula can have a positive effect on adolescent health outcomes (Young, Leger, & Blanchard, 2013). For example, health education leading to greater mental health literacy (MHL) would allow more recognition of disorders. In mental health situations, "[o]nce depression is recognized, help can make a difference for 80% of people who are affected, allowing them to get back to their regular activities." (Canadian Mental Health Association, 2014, § How does it impact youth?, para. 4).

Parents, too, are health educators and have a major role to play in adolescent health literacy and learning. Parental modelling and attitudes concerning health behaviours can have a significant effect on adolescent health behaviours (Gavin, Catalano, David-Ferdon, Gloppen, & Markham, 2010). Parents act as models for healthy eating and exercise, responsible alcohol use, and managing stress, for example. Adolescents whose parents smoke (Maggi et al., 2014) or use cannabis (Degenhardt et al., 2010) are more likely to engage in these health-risk behaviours. Parental support is an important factor in helping adolescents attain good health (Viner et al., 2012). Beets, Cardinal, and Alderman (2010) reported that the professional literature shows that parents are (a) role models in reinforcing and advocating for adolescent health-promoting and health-risk behaviours and (b) a "primary source of health information and education" for adolescents (p. 2). Adult allies of all kinds are invaluable to support adolescent health literacy and learning.

AUDIENCE FOR THE BOOK

Adolescent Health Literacy and Learning, then, is directed to a wide audience of university students, practicing health educators and practitioners, family members, and policy makers. Both undergraduate and graduate students in health and health-related disciplines —

such as physical education, medicine, nursing, social work, and youth care — will discover in this book insights into adolescent health literacy and learning. Inservice teachers and coaches in schools and in the community will add to their existing knowledge and experience concerning middle school and high school students' health behaviours. Likewise, parents, grandparents, and other adolescent caregivers will find ideas. Policy makers, too, are an audience we hope will engage with the authors in this book as adolescent health literacy and learning needs are specific and important societal needs. Finally, citizens in general will find in this book a variety of readings on today's young adult health learners. We recommend this book to all of you who touch the lives of adolescents.

OVERVIEW OF THE BOOK

Fostering adolescent health literacy and learning in a variety of educational contexts — both within and beyond the school — needs up-to-date approaches and theoretical foundations that are specific to adolescents. Our book offers this focus. *Adolescent Health Literacy and Learning* has four chapters on topics of general interest including adolescent health literacy concepts, theoretical models, and use of engaging novels that feature health topics and six chapters with a more specific focus.

General Topic Chapters

In this chapter (Why Focus on Adolescent Health Literacy and Learning?), we offer an introduction to the concept of adolescent health, adolescent health literacy, and adolescent learning and the importance of education and parents to address adolescent health literacy development.

In chapter 2 (Definitions of Adolescent Health Literacy: A Systematic Review and Critical Appraisal), Malloy-Weir provides a conceptual overview of definitions of health literacy that have been applied to youth populations by reviewing 30 academic articles that purport to address adolescent health literacy, often without clear definitions. The author then makes a case for the importance of addressing the adolescent context with appropriate benchmarks in order to address their health literacy needs and to develop a standard health literacy vocabulary for practitioners and researchers working with adolescent populations.

In chapter 9 (Addressing Girls' Health Literacy and Learning with Young Adult 'Problem' Novels), Begoray, Banister, and Jaswal suggest ways to choose and use young adult novels to introduce health and wellness topics to girls. These so-called problem novels show adolescent girls struggling with challenging health issues such as fatal illness, death, bullying, drug and alcohol abuse, prejudice, isolation, eating disorders, and date rape. Adolescents are drawn to these novels despite, or even because of, their unsettling topics. The authors review 11 novels by, first, providing plot summaries, then discussing the health topics that are featured in these novels and providing further information and resources for readers. Finally, the authors provide writing, visual representing, and talking activities that might be used by a teacher with a class of adolescents or by a health practitioner who was using these novels for health education with a single adolescent.

Finally, in the last chapter (chapter 10, Looking Back and Looking Ahead), we discuss the major themes of the book, drawing together threads from each chapter. We then suggest what the future might hold for the field of adolescent health literacy and learning by identifying and discussing several trends.

Specific Focus Chapters

The six more specific chapters of *Adolescent Health Literacy and Learning* focus on one or more of three major topics: media and technology, gender, and mental health. These themes frequently overlap within articles; that is, one article may offer insight into, for example, both gender and media (e.g., chapter 5, Banister and Begoray, Teaching Middle Adolescents to Critically Reflect on the Interaction of Gender with Health; chapter 6, Wharf Higgins and Bellows Riecken, Fast Food and Fitness: Gendered Health Literacy Needs of High School Students). In addition to these major topics, authors discuss such diverse topics as youth suicide (chapter 8, Ranahan, Mental Health Literacies in Youth Work Practice with Adolescents), graphic novels (chapter 3, Begoray and Fu, Reading *Chasing Adland*: Middle Years' Students in Pursuit of Critical Media Health Literacy), and MHL for Indigenous teens (chapter 7, Marshall, Integrating Culture to Enhance Mental Health Literacy among Aboriginal Youth).

Media and Technology

Current health literacy learning approaches are often out of touch with today's adolescents. Ghaddar, Valerio, Garcia, and Hansen (2012) recommended the use of online sources such as Medline Plus in high school health curricula, citing the prevalence of online health information seeking by adolescents. Teachers find technology use is motivating for adolescents, allowing students to use skills more generally associated with out-of-school activities (e.g., creating websites and video games) in the classroom and to bridge interests in popular culture (e.g., graphic novels) with more traditional school activities.

Media and computer technology's darker face as the powerful tool of commercial advertisers is another topic that needs to be discussed with adolescents. Begoray and Fu in chapter 3 present a research study that investigated the behaviours and opinions of middle school students and their teacher who were involved in using a graphic novel to learn about advertising's impact on adolescent health and wellness. (The comic book style graphic novel had been written by another group of adolescents specifically for a peer-age audience.) This group of middle school readers was engaged by the novel's story and drawings. They also showed evidence during the in-class lessons and in follow-up interviews of critical thinking about the impact of the media on their health. The authors conclude that both creating and reading graphic novels has the potential to help adolescents become more health literate.

Beer and Begoray in chapter 4 examine the media interactions of wealthy high school students in Burma/Myanmar. These Grade 10 students both consumed and created websites and blogs about mental health as part of an interdisciplinary unit of study. They were particularly interested in the impact of social media on their sense of mental wellbeing. While some students proved to be anxious about media influences, others were more optimistic. One group even showed evidence of taking control of media and, thus, controlling its influence on their mental health. The authors conclude that context is a particularly important factor influencing health literacy for adolescents. Students in affluent circumstances in a poverty-stricken country run by a military dictatorship still, like their western adolescent counterparts, are learning to cope with the power of the online media.

Gender

Authors in this book writing on gender understand it as "a social construct, a multidimensional determinant of health that intersects with culturally prescribed and experienced dimensions of femininity and masculinity" (Bottorff, Oliffe, & Kelly, 2012, p. 435). Banister and Begoray in chapter 5 examine the gendered effects of advertising on middle years' students. They developed lessons to teach groups of girls and boys who worked in small gender-specific groups how to create video advertisements and then explored how these students portrayed themselves using stick-puppet avatars. Interviews revealed how these boys and girls portrayed masculinity and femininity visually and how they discussed their choices verbally. The authors conclude that the media exerts strong influence on young adolescents' understanding of what it means to be a boy or girl and that this understanding needs to be taken into account by health literacy educators and researchers, especially those working in the area of media health literacy.

Wharf Higgins and Bellows Riecken in chapter 6 present their findings on gender influences on choice of nutrition and exercise amongst male and female adolescents in a health-promoting secondary school. All students were critical of the efforts of health education classes to give realistic advice on the sedentary effects of their increasing involvement in screen time, but the researchers also found that there were indeed differences in boys' and girls' health literacy concerning exercise and healthy eating. The authors conclude that in order to raise levels of health literacy we need to take into account the gendered understandings of high school adolescents.

Mental Health

Physical and Health Education Canada (2014) reported that "[t]he mental and emotional health and well-being of youth is a serious and underserved Canadian health issue. At any given time, 15 per cent of our young people are affected by mental health issues, with 70 per cent of all psychiatric disorders emerging in adolescence" (para. 2). Rates of suicide are especially alarming as the second most frequent cause of death amongst adolescents in Canada with only accidental death as a more common cause of mortality. In the United States, "[j]ust over 20 percent (or 1 in 5) children [up to age 18], either currently or at some point during their life, have had a seriously debilitating mental disorder" (National Institute of Mental Health, n.d., para. 1) including those that lead to suicide.

In this book in chapter 8, Ranahan presents a newly conceptualized definition of MHL that draws upon examples from her research with youth workers who deal with suicidal adolescents. Ranahan suggests that MHL needs to move beyond its current definition as the ability to merely recognize mental disorders. Rather, it needs to include both critical and social literacies such as the ability to develop caring relationships, use nonverbal as well as verbal communication strategies and the ability to take action, such as challenging authority when necessary. Ranahan's work on the MHL of youth workers extends to adolescents themselves who have wisdom about mental health and whose ideas need to be more fully acknowledged and integrated into theoretical concepts.

In chapter 7, Marshall examines MHL and learning in Aboriginal youth populations. Aboriginal youth have much higher rates of unmet mental health care needs than do non-Aboriginal adolescents. For example, the leading cause of death in this population is suicide. In addition, their numbers are growing more rapidly than the general adolescent population. Marshall suggests that education has a major role to play in using cultural factors, especially in integrating cultural safety into MHL programs. In particular, Aboriginal youth need to be engaged and empowered to improve their MHL. Likewise, adult allies of these youth need higher levels of Aboriginal MHL in order to help effectively.

All these authors agree: *adolescent health literacy and learning matters*. It matters for adolescents now and in their future. Various themes emerge from these chapters that will be discussed in chapter 10, Looking Back and Looking Ahead.

Structure of the Chapters

Each chapter in this book begins with *Focusing Questions*. We encourage you to pause before beginning the chapter by thinking about your own responses to these questions. Effective learning involves accessing one's prior knowledge and background experiences about the topic. You may want to discuss your responses with others and/or write down your answers. Each chapter ends with *Questions for Discussion, Reflection, and Writing*. Once you have completed reading the chapter, these questions encourage thinking about learning in order to consolidate your new understanding. Talking with other readers, reflecting individually, and writing are three ways to integrate new knowledge with previous knowledge.

Features of the Book

Features of this book besides the chapters include: Biographical List of Contributors, List of Online Resources, and an Index. In the Biographical List of Contributors, each contributing author has provided a brief summary of their position and academic interests. In addition, email addresses are available so you can contact each author if you have questions or comments. The List of Online Resources, found at the end of each chapter, gives website links that have been provided by the contributing authors as recommendations for further reading on the topic of their chapter. Finally, the Index will help you to locate many of this book's important topics.

Acknowledgments

We acknowledge with gratitude the many contributors to this volume. They are passionate about adolescents and gave generously of their time to write chapters. You can learn more about them in the Biographical List of Contributors.

We particularly thank Dr. Irv Rootman for his generosity in serving as the author of the Foreword. Dr. Rootman has written many Forewords for a number of scholars who have authored or edited books on health literacy including *Health Literacy in Context: International Perspectives* (Begoray, Gillis, & Rowlands, 2012). We note with pride that Dr. Rootman is the recent recipient (2014) of Doctor of Law, *Honoris causa* from the University of Victoria, Canada, for his national and international contributions to the field of health literacy.

We are grateful for the patience and skill of Shari Yore, our copy and style editor. She was efficient, patient, and helpful as we brought together the sometimes disparate voices of this book to form a coherent whole and to make it more than the sum of its parts.

To Nova Science Inc., who have once again given a place in their catalog to us as health literacy scholars and researchers, we acknowledge your belief in our collective work.

Finally, to the adolescents we work with and the many others touched by the work of health researchers and educators, thank you for your voices as they appear in this book. And to the others still waiting for better adolescent health literacy and learning opportunities, we hope this volume will inspire our readers to take up your cause.

Questions for Discussion, Reflection, and Writing

1. What chapters are you most interested in reading? Why?
2. What are your goals in reading this book? What understanding do you hope to gain?
3. Why are adolescents particularly of importance to you and to the authors of this book?

List of Online Resources

- Nemours: Teens Health – http://kidshealth.org/teen/expert/
- Johns Hopkins Bloomberg School of Public Health: Center for Adolescent Health – http://www.jhsph.edu/research/centers-and-institutes/center-for-adolescent-health/

References

Anderman, E. M. (2002). School effects on psychological outcomes during adolescence. *Journal of Educational Psychology, 94,* 795–809.

Anderman, E. M., Sinatra, G. M., & Gray, D. (2012). The challenges of teaching and learning about science in the twenty-first century: Exploring the abilities and constraints of adolescent learners. *Studies in Science Education, 48*(1), 89–117.

Banister, E., Begoray, D., & Daly, L. K. (2011). Responding to adolescent women's reproductive health concerns: Empowering clients through health literacy. *Health Care for Women International, 32*(4), 344–354. doi:10.1080/07399332.2010.536603

Beets, M. W., Cardinal, B. J., & Alderman, B. L. (2010). Parental social support and the physical activity-related behaviors of youth: A review. *Health Education & Behavior, 37*(5), 621–644.

Begoray, D., Cimon, M., & Wharf Higgins, J. (2010). *Mediating health: The powerful role of media as adolescent health literacy educator*. Hauppauge, NY: Nova Science.

Begoray, D., Gillis, D., & Rowlands, G. (Eds.). (2012). *Health literacy in context: International perspectives*. Hauppauge, NY: Nova Science.

Blanton, W., & Wood, D. (2009). The case for improving adolescent literacy instruction. In K. Woods & W. Blanton, *Literacy instruction for adolescents: Research based practice* (pp. 1–12). New York, NY: Guilford Press.

Blum, R. W., Bastos, F. I. P. M., Kabiru, C., & Le, L. C. (2012). Adolescent health in the 21st century. *The Lancet, 379*, 1567–1568.

Bottorff, J. L., Oliffe, J. L., & Kelly, M. T. (2012). The gender(s) in the room. *Qualitative Health Research, 22*(4), 435–440.

British Columbia Ministry of Education. (2007). *Planning 10: Integrated resource package 2007.* Victoria, BC: Author. Retrieved from http://www.bced.gov.bc.ca/irp/ pdfs/ health_career_education/2007planning10.pdf

Canadian Mental Health Association. (2014). *Fast facts about mental illness*. Ottawa, ON: Author. Retrieved from http://www.cmha.ca/media/fast-facts-about-mental-illness/#.VPow7PnF-GE

Chinn, C. A., & Malhotra, B. A. (2002). Epistemologically authentic inquiry in schools: A theoretical framework for evaluating inquiry tasks. *Science Education, 86*(2), 175–218.

Degenhardt, L., Coffey, C., Carlin, J. B., Swift, W., Moore, E., & Patton, G. C. (2010). Outcomes of occasional cannabis use in adolescence: 10-year follow-up study in Victoria, Australia. *British Journal of Psychiatry, 196*(4), 290–295.

Gavin, L. E., Catalano, R. F., David-Ferdon, C., Gloppen, K. M., & Markham, C. M. (2010). A review of positive youth development programs that promote adolescent sexual and reproductive health. *Journal of Adolescent Health, 46*(3), S75–S91.

Ghaddar, S. F., Valerio, M. A., Garcia, C. M., & Hansen, I. (2012). Adolescent health literacy: The importance of credible sources for online health information. *Journal of School Health, 82*(1), 28–36.

Gray, S. L., Culpepper, C. L., & Welsh, D. P. (2012). Adolescence. In V. S. Ramachandran (Ed.), *Encyclopedia of human behavior* (2nd ed.). London, England: Academic Press.

Guttmacher Institute. (2014, May). *American teens' sexual and reproductive health* (Fact Sheet). New York, NY: Author. Retrieved from http://www. guttmacher.org/pubs/FB-ATSRH.pdf

Health Canada. (2012). *Canadian alcohol and drug use monitoring survey*. Ottawa, ON: Author. Retrieved from http://www.hc-sc.gc.ca/hc-ps/drugs-drogues/stat/_2012/ summary-sommaire-eng.php

Kaufman, M. (2006). Role of adolescent development in the transition process. *Progress in Transplantation, 16*(4), 286–290.

Kolbe, L. (2005). A framework for school health programs in the 21st century. *Journal of School Health, 75*(6), 226–228.

Lê, F., Roux, A., & Morgenstern, H. (2012). Effects of child and adolescent health on educational progress. *Social Sciences and Medicine, 76*, 57–66.

Maggi, S., Lovato, C. Y., Hill, E. M., Johnson, J. L., Ratner, P. A., & Shoveller, J. A. (2012). Adolescents' perceptions of parental influences on their smoking behavior: A content analysis. *Youth & Society, 46*(1), 132–149.

Manganello, J. (2008). Health literacy and adolescents: A framework and agenda for future research. *Health Education Research, 23*(5), 840–847.

Marcus, M., & Westra, H. (2012). Mental health literacy in Canadian young adults: Results of a national survey. *Canadian Journal of Community Mental Health, 31*(1), 1–15.

Matthews, N., Kilgour, L., Christian, P., Mori, K., & Hill, D. M. (2014). Understanding, evidencing, and promoting adolescent well-being: An emerging agenda for schools. *Youth & Society*. Advance online publication. doi:10.1177/0044118X13513590

National Institute of Mental Health. (n.d.). *Any disorder among children*. Bethesda, MD: Author. Retrieved from http://www.nimh.nih.gov/health/ statistics/prevalence/any-disorder-among-children.shtml

Nutbeam, D. (2000). Health literacy as a public health goal: A challenge for contemporary health education and communication strategies into the 21st century. *Health Promotion International, 15*(3), 259–267.

Paakkari, L., & Paakkari, O. (2012). Health literacy as a learning outcome in schools. *Health Education, 112*(2), 133–152.

Partnership for 21st Century Skills. (2011). *Framework for 21st century learning*. Washington, DC: Author. Retrieved from http://www.p21.org/ storage/documents/ 1.__p21_framework_2-pager.pdf

Perry, E. L. (2014). Health literacy in adolescents: An integrative review. *Journal for Specialists in Pediatric Nursing, 19*(3), 210–218.

Persson, L., & Haraldsson, K. (2013). Health promotion in Swedish schools: School managers' views. *Health Promotion International.* Advance online publication. doi:10.1093/heapro/dat073

Physical and Health Education Canada. (2014). *Youth mental health*. Ottawa, ON: Author. Retrieved from http://www.phecanada.ca/programs/youth-mental-health

Price, M., & Dalgleish, J. (2013). Help-seeking among Indigenous Australian adolescents. Exploring attitudes, behaviours and barriers. *Youth Studies Australia, 32*(1), 10–18.

Reeve, J. (2009). Why teachers adopt a controlling motivating style toward students and how they can become more autonomy supportive. *Educational Psychologist, 44*(3), 159–175.

Rootman, I., & Gordon-El-Bihbety, D. (2008). *A vision for a health literate Canada: Report of the expert panel on health literacy.* Ottawa, ON: Canadian Public Health Association. Retrieved from http://www.cpha.ca/ uploads/portals/h-l/report_e.pdf

Rothman, R., Yin, S., Mulvaney, S., Co, J., Homer, C., & Lannon, C. (2009). Health literacy and quality: Focus on chronic illness care and patient safety. *Pediatrics, 124*, s315–s326.

Smart, K. A., Parker, R. S., Lampert, J., & Sulo, S. (2012). Speaking up: Teens voice their health information needs. *Journal of School Nursing, 28*(5), 379–388.

Suleiman, A. B., & Brindis, C. D. (2014). Adolescent school-based sex education: Using developmental neuroscience to guide new directions for policy and practice. *Sexuality Research and Social Policy, 11*(2), 137–152.

United Nations Fund for Population Activities. (2011). *The state of the world population*. New York, NY: United Nations Population Fund.

Van Cleave, J., Gortmaker, S. L., & Perrin, J. M. (2010). Dynamics of obesity and chronic health conditions among children and youth. *JAMA, 303*(7), 623–630.

Viner, R. M., Ozer, E. M., Denny, S., Marmot, M., Resnick, M., Fatusi, A., & Currie, C. (2012). Adolescence and the social determinants of health. *The Lancet, 379*(9826), 1641–1652.

Wharf Higgins, J., Begoray, D., & MacDonald, M. (2009). A social ecological conceptual framework for understanding adolescent health literacy in the health education classroom. *American Journal of Community Psychology, 44*(3–4), 350–362.

World Health Organization. (2012). *Health education: Theoretical concepts, effective strategies and core competencies.* Cairo, Egypt: Regional Office for the Eastern Mediterranean. Retrieved from http://applications.emro. who.int/dsaf/ EMRPUB_2012_EN_1362.pdf

World Health Organization. (2014). *Adolescents: Health risks and solutions* (Fact Sheet No. 345). Geneva, Switzerland: Author. Retrieved from http://www.who.int/ mediacentre/factsheets/fs345/en

Young, I., Leger, L., & Blanchard, C. (2013). Health-promoting schools: Working in partnership to address global needs. A collaboration leading to the production of practical tools for practitioners. *Global Health Promotion, 20*(Suppl. 4), 122–127.

Zimmet, P. Z. (2011). The growing pandemic of type 2 diabetes: A crucial need for prevention and improved detection. *Medicographia*, *33*(1), 15–21.

In: Adolescent Health Literacy and Learning
Editors: D. L. Begoray and E. M. Banister
ISBN: 978-1-63482-897-0

Chapter 2

DEFINITIONS OF ADOLESCENT HEALTH LITERACY: A SYSTEMATIC REVIEW AND CRITICAL APPRAISAL

Leslie Malloy-Weir*
Health Policy Program Doctoral Student, McMaster University, Ontario, Canada

ABSTRACT

Previous reviews of definitions of health literacy have sought to identify, analyze and, in some cases, classify different definitions derived from a variety of sources. While these reviews have been helpful for understanding how health literacy has been defined, the perceived relevance of any one or more definitions to adolescents is unknown. This chapter systematically identifies, and then critically appraises, definitions of health literacy used in adolescent research. Based on the findings, an argument is made for the development of definitions that explicate how health literacy in adolescents differs from health literacy in children, adults, and seniors. An argument is also made for the development of benchmarks to: (1) facilitate the development of measures of health literacy that are appropriate for use in adolescent populations; (2) inform the development, implementation, and evaluation of efforts to promote health literacy in adolescents; and (3) allow parents, researchers, teachers, policymakers, health practitioners, and members from the community to speak a common language when communicating about health literacy in adolescents.

Keywords: adolescents, health literacy, definitions

Focusing Questions

1. What is your definition of adolescent health literacy?
2. Why are definitions of adolescent health literacy important in health promotion, policy, teaching, and research?

* Correspondence to (email): malloylj@mcmaster.ca.

The World Health Organization (WHO, 2015) defines adolescence as "the period in human growth and development that occurs after childhood and before adulthood, from ages 10 to 19" (para. 1). During this period of rapid growth, adolescents "are not fully capable of understanding complex concepts, or the relationship between behavior and consequences, or the degree of control they have or can have over health decision making" (para. 4). As such, adolescents are at risk for engaging in, or developing, risky behaviours that may carry over into adulthood or lead to intentional or unintentional injuries.

The promotion of health literacy has been identified as one way to prevent negative health outcomes in adolescents (Sanders, Shaw, Guez, Baur, & Rudd, 2009) and prepare adolescents to be active participants in their health care (Diamond, Saintonge, August, & Azrack, 2011). Models for health literacy and child health promotion (i.e., up to the age of 18 years) have also been developed that specify roles for health systems, the patient care environment, the educational system, and community systems (Sanders et al., 2009). For each to fulfil these roles, an understanding of adolescent health literacy is required. Such understanding is needed for measurement-related purposes and to avoid misunderstandings when communicating about adolescent health literacy.

Previous reviews of definitions of health literacy have sought to identify, analyze and, in some cases, classify definitions of health literacy (Berkman, Davis, & McCormack, 2010; Peerson & Saunders, 2009; Rudd, McCray, & Nutbeam, 2012; Sorensen et al., 2012). While these reviews are helpful for understanding how health literacy has been defined, the perceived relevance of any one or more of these definitions for adolescents is unknown. This chapter, therefore, begins by identifying how adolescent health literacy — or health literacy in adolescents — has been defined in the academic literature. A critical appraisal of the definitions identified follows. The implications of the findings for efforts to promote and measure health literacy in adolescents are then discussed.

Summary of Methods

A systematic review (Petticrew & Roberts, 2006) and critical appraisal of the literature (Hughes, 1996) was conducted for definitions of adolescent health literacy and health literacy in adolescent research. A search of electronic databases (i.e., Medline, Embase, ERIC, CINAHL) took place on June 24, 2014, using *adolescent health literacy* as a keyword; it returned a total of 38 articles. After de-duplication, 30 articles remained, which were then searched for definitions of *adolescent health literacy* or *health literacy*.

A matrix (Miles & Huberman, 1994) was used to display and compare definitions extracted from the literature. Definitions that were identical in wording were grouped in the same row in the matrix; definitions that differed in wording were assigned their own row. This allowed for a numerical count of how often any given definition of adolescent health literacy was used in the academic literature.

Critical appraisal of adolescent health literacy definitions involved asking two questions of each definition. The first question — *Are there words in the definition that are vague or ambiguous?* — helped to identify words that could be interpreted differently. The second question — *What assumptions underlie the definition?* — helped to identify any implied or explicit relationships or beliefs about the definition that may not be fully supported by empirical research. The answers to these questions, along with analytic comments related to measurement or use of the definition in policy, practice, research, or teaching, were entered into the matrix.

RESULTS

How Has Adolescent Health Literacy Been Defined in the Academic Literature?

None of the 30 articles reviewed contained a definition of adolescent health literacy despite explicit mention of adolescent health literacy in the titles of five (Ghaddar, Valerio, Garcia, & Hansen, 2012; Gray, Klein, Noyce, Sesselberg, & Cantrill, 2005; Massey et al., 2013; Skopelja, Whipple, & Richwine, 2008; Wharf Higgins, Begoray, & MacDonald, 2009). Nevertheless, 12 articles contained one or more definitions of health literacy in general. As shown in the Appendix, 15 different definitions of health literacy were extracted from the literature. Ratzan and Parker's (2000) definition of health literacy — "the capacity of individuals to obtain, process, and understand basic health information and services needed to make appropriate health decisions" (p. vi) — was provided in four articles. Rootman and Gordon-El-Bihbety's (2008) definition — "the ability to access, understand, evaluate and communicate information as a way to promote, maintain and improve health in a variety of settings across the lifecourse" (p. 11) — was provided in two articles. The 13 remaining definitions appeared only once in the articles.

What Are the Similarities and Differences across Definitions?

Row-by-row comparison of the wording used in definitions listed in the Appendix revealed some similarities and differences. Similarities included the specification of abilities, skills, or capacities believed to comprise health literacy. While these abilities, skills, and capacities varied across definitions, they explicitly, or implicitly, were attributed to individuals. Other similarities related to context. In three definitions, context(s) relevant to health literacy were specified; however, they were variable across definitions in terms of their scope. Narrow contexts included "the health care environment" (Gray et al., 2005, p. e2). Broad contexts included "everyday life" (Wharf Higgins et al., 2009, p. 352) and "a variety of settings across the life course" (Rootman & Gordon-El-Bihbety, 2008, p. 11).

Possible Interpretations of Definitions

In column three of the Appendix, a summary of the critical appraisal of health literacy definitions is provided. This summary illustrates how different interpretations of health literacy in adolescents may arise through the presence of vague or ambiguous wording. It is unclear, for example, what authors mean by the words *obtain* (Peterson, Cooper, & Laird, 2001; Ratzan & Parker, 2000; Vardavas, Kondilis, Patelarou, Akrivos, & Falagas, 2009), *process* (Ratzan & Parker, 2000; Vardavas et al., 2009), *use* (Gray et al., 2005; Paek, Reber, & Lariscy, 2011; Peterson et al., 2001), and *basic health information* (Peterson et al., 2001; Ratzan & Parker, 2000; Vardavas et al., 2009). The source, credibility, type, applicability, and acceptability of the information that was mentioned in 11 definitions (Gray et al., 2005; Massey et al., 2013; Paek et al., 2011; Peterson et al., 2001; Ratzan & Parker, 2000; Rootman & Gordon-El-Bihbety, 2008; Vardavas et al., 2009; Wharf Higgins et al., 2009; Wu et al., 2010) is also unclear. Terms such as *required* (Vardavas et al., 2009), *appropriate* (Ratzan & Parker, 2000), *sound* (Kickbush as cited in Wharf Higgins et al., 2009), *understand* (Gray et al., 2005; Peterson et al., 2001; Ratzan & Parker, 2000; Skopelja et al., 2008; Vardavas, 2009; Wu et al., 2010), and *evaluate* (Rootman & Gordon-El-Bihbety, 2008) are also problematic because it is not clear who determines what is required, appropriate, or sound for adolescents or whose understanding(s) or evaluation(s) are valued.

In nine of the definitions listed in the Appendix, the criteria that must be met, or the threshold at which health literacy is achieved in adolescents, are not clear. In three definitions, criteria are provided. These criteria include when an individual is "able to understand and apply health information in ways that allow them to take more control over their health" (Wu et al., 2010, p. 445), "when the skills and the ability of those requiring health information and services are aligned with the demand and complexity of information and services" (Massey et al., 2013, p. 342), and when a person is "able to use health concepts and information generatively, applying information to novel situations" (Paek et al., 2011, p. 133). These criteria are, however, non-overlapping.

Underlying assumptions that may not be fully supported by empirical research are present in seven definitions (Gray et al., 2005; Paek et al., 2011; Peterson et al., 2001; Ratzan & Parker, 2001; Rootman & Gordon-El-Bihbety, 2008; Vardavas et al., 2009; Wu et al., 2010). The definition provided by Wu and colleagues (2010), for example, implies that a relationship exists between adolescents' ability to understand and apply health information and their ability to take control over their health (e.g., by changing health behaviours or living conditions). Support for the need to be cautious about assumptions that link health literacy with health behaviours can be found in a study of adolescents in Taiwan (Chang, 2011). In that study, adolescents with high and low health literacy (as indicated by the c-sTOFHLAd [Chinese short version of the Test of Functional Health Literacy in Adolescents]) differed significantly in terms of some health promoting behaviours (i.e., nutrition and interpersonal relations), but not others (i.e., exercise, stress management, health responsibility, and self-actualisations). The author stated that, "[I]n Chinese culture, most adolescents are under family domination and partially or fully rely on their parents to make health-related decisions until they get married" (Chang, 2009, p. 195). This statement provides a clear example of the importance of context in understanding health literacy in adolescents.

DISCUSSION

The findings of this review both support, and add to, findings previously reported in the literature. Consistent with previous reviews of general definitions of health literacy (e.g., Berkman et al., 2010; Sorensen et al., 2012), this review found a lack of agreement over the definition(s) of health literacy that are perceived as relevant to adolescents. This lack of agreement poses challenges for policymakers, researchers, health care practitioners, and teachers who jointly seek to promote health literacy in adolescents but define and interpret it differently. This finding also raises questions about which definition(s) of health literacy should be adopted for use in adolescent populations, the criteria on which this decision should be based, and who should be involved in the decision-making process.

While consideration of context may be helpful for guiding the adoption of any given definition(s), only three definitions identified in this review specified contexts relevant to health literacy. These contexts were, however, non-overlapping. Adolescence is situated within the context of human development and is a period in life that is distinctly different from childhood, adulthood, and old age. As such, definitions of adolescent health literacy are needed to clearly distinguish how it differs from health literacy in children and adults. Differentiating health literacy in this manner would help foster the development of measures and health literacy-based interventions that are more appropriate for adolescent populations.

The findings of this review also demonstrate some of the potentially problematic assumptions inherent in definitions of health literacy used in adolescent research. Policymakers should be cautious about acting on assumptions that link health literacy to health behaviours or health decisions given that adolescents are not fully capable of understanding "the relationship between behavior and consequences, or the degree of control they have or can have over health decision making" (WHO, 2015, para. 4). Action on unsupported assumptions may lead to the neglect of other factors, such as parents (Chang, 2011), that influence health behaviours and health decision making in adolescents.

Last, the definitions identified in this review contained vague and ambiguous wording, leaving them open to varying, and potentially conflicting, interpretations. While the flexibility to develop, adopt, and interpret any given definition(s) of health literacy may be welcomed or encouraged by policymakers and researchers seeking to promote health literacy in adolescents, the same flexibility may undermine efforts to develop, implement, and evaluate efforts to promote health literacy in adolescents — particularly when those involved define and interpret it differently. To this end, the adoption of stipulative definitions (Hughes, 1996), in which the precise meaning of key words is stipulated by researchers and policymakers, may help to reduce misunderstandings and increase clarity and precision.

Another way to gain clarity and precision would be to develop benchmarks, such as those suggested by Sanders et al. (2009), for the promotion of health literacy in children and adolescents. Reference to these benchmarks in definitions of health literacy would help to make their meaning less abstract and more concrete. Beyond the added clarity, benchmarks would encourage the development of specific health literacy skills in adolescents (i.e., oral, prose/document, numeracy, system navigation skills) by a specific age (e.g., 10, 14, and 18 years). This type of specification would make it easier to develop, implement, and evaluate the effectiveness of initiatives to promote health literacy in adolescents. It would facilitate the development of measures of health literacy for use in adolescent populations. The use of benchmarks would also allow policymakers, parents, and members from different sectors (i.e., health systems, community systems, the educational system, and the patient care environment) to speak a common language when talking about health literacy in adolescents.

LIMITATIONS

Some limitations concerning bias exist with this review (Petticrew & Roberts, 2006). First, the search was limited to English language articles. Reviews in other languages are needed to determine a wider prevalence of, and interpretations for, definitions of adolescent health literacy. Second, interpretations beyond those identified by the author are possible. Another limitation is the small number of articles returned in the search, due to the use of *adolescent health literacy* as a search term. Future reviews that are less restrictive in regard to the search terms used could generate a larger number of definitions for analysis.

CONCLUSION

Prior to this review, the perceived relevance of definitions of health literacy for adolescents was unknown. While some of the findings from this review overlap with those of previous reviews of general definitions of health literacy, they suggest a need for the development of definitions of health literacy that are specific to the adolescent context. Definitions of adolescent health literacy are needed not only to develop measures of adolescent health literacy but also to inform the development of health literacy-based initiatives that are appropriate for this population.

Questions for Discussion, Reflection, and Writing

3. What criterion, or criteria, should be used to guide the adoption of any given definitions(s) of health literacy for use in adolescent populations?
4. Who should be involved in the adoption and interpretation of any definition(s) of health literacy used in adolescent populations?
5. What health literacy skills should be developed in adolescents who are 10, 14, and 18 years of age?

List of Online Resources

- World Health Organization: Adolescent Health – http://www.who.int/topics/adolescent_ health/en/
- Health Literacy and Child Health Promotion: Implications for Research, Clinical Care, and Public Policy – http:// pediatrics.aappublications.org/content/124/Supplement_3/S306.full.pdf

APPENDIX.

Definitions of health literacy used in adolescent research and analytical comments with implications for measurement, policy, research, and teaching

Row	Definitions and their source*	Analytical comments
1	"Health literacy is defined as the capacity of individuals to **obtain, interpret,** and **understand basic health information and services**, and the competence to **use** such information and services **in ways that enhance health**." Peterson et al. (2001, p. 140, citing Joint Committee on National Health Education Standards, 1995)	Unclear what is meant by or what constitutes *obtain, process, interpret, understand, basic health information and services, use, ways that enhance health* in adolescents. Unclear whose understanding is valued. Implies that a link exists between (a) obtaining, interpreting, and understanding of basic health information and services and (b) the enhancement of health in adolescents. The threshold at which health literacy is achieved in adolescents is not clear.
2	"The degree to which individuals have the capacity to **obtain, process**, and understand **basic health information and services** needed to make **appropriate health decisions**." (Ratzan & Parker, 2000, p. vi) Brown, Teufel, & Birch (2007, p. 8, citing Healthy People, 2010) Skopelja et al. (2008, p. 106, citing Healthy People, 2010) Paek et al. (2011, p. 132, citing Ratzan & Parker, 2000) Ghaddar et al. (2012, p. 28, citing Nielsen-Bohlman et al., 2004)	Unclear what is meant by or what constitutes *obtain, process, understand, basic health information and services, appropriate health decisions* in adolescents. Unclear whose understanding is valued. Unclear who decides (a) what *basic health information and services* are *needed* by adolescents or (b) what type(s) or kind(s) of *health decisions* are *appropriate* for adolescents. Unclear whether or not the phrase *needed to make appropriate health decisions* (a) refers to the basic health information and services preceding it, and/or (b) implies that, in order for adolescents to be health literate, they need to make *appropriate health decisions*. Implies that a link exists between (a) obtaining, processing, and understanding of basic health information and services and (b) the making of appropriate health decisions by adolescents. The threshold at which health literacy is achieved in adolescents is not clear.
3	"the degree of ability to **obtain, process**, and understand the **basic health information and services** ***required*** to make appropriate health decisions." Vardavas et al. (2009, p. 179, citing Nutbeam & Kickbusch, 2000; and Gazamararian et al., 2003)	A modified version of the Ratzan and Parker (2000) definition that appears in column 1, row 2. Analytic comments in column 3, row 2 apply to this definition with one exception: unclear who decides *what basic health information and services* are ***required*** by adolescents.

Appendix. (Continued)

Row	Definitions and their source*	Analytical comments
4	"the skills which determine the motivation and ability of individuals to **access, understand**, and **use information in ways that promote and maintain good health**." Gray et al. (2005, p. e2, citing WHO, 1999)	Unclear what is meant by and what constitutes *access, understand, use, information, in ways that promote and maintain good health* in adolescents. Unclear whose understanding is valued. The skills that determine motivation and ability of adolescents are unspecified. This definition is different from others in that it has a motivation component. The definition implies that skills determine the motivation and ability of adolescents. It is possible, however, that the relationship(s) between (a) skills and (b) motivation and ability may be bi-directional in adolescents. Implies that a relationship exists between (a) accessing, understanding, and using of information and (b) the promotion and maintenance of good health. The threshold at which health literacy is achieved in adolescents is not clear.
5	"constellation of skills, including the ability to perform **basic reading and numerical tasks** required to **function in the health care environment**." Gray et al. (2005, p. e2, citing AMA, 1999)	Unclear what is meant by or what constitutes *basic reading and numerical tasks* and *function in the health care environment* in adolescents. Unclear if the *constellation of skills* is fully, or only partially, specified in the definition. Unclear who determines what *basic reading and numerical tasks* are required by adolescents to *function in the health care environment.* Implies a relationship between *basic reading and numerical tasks* and adolescents' functioning in the health care environment. The threshold at which health literacy is achieved in adolescents is not clear.
6	"The ability to **make sound health decisions** in the context of everyday life … It is a critical empowerment strategy to increase people's **control over their health**, their ability to **seek out information** and their ability to **take responsibility**." Wharf Higgins et al. (2009, p. 352, citing Kickbusch, 2007)	This definition is different from others in that it specifies context. Unclear what is meant by or what constitutes *sound health decisions, control over their health, seek out, information, take responsibility* in adolescents. Unclear who determines what *sound health decisions* are for adolescents. Implies that adolescents are autonomous in their health decision making. The threshold at which health literacy is achieved in adolescents is not clear.

Row	Definitions and their source*	Analytical comments
7	"The ability to **access, understand, evaluate** and **communicate information** as a **way** to **promote, maintain and improve health** in a variety of settings across the lifecourse." Wharf Higgins et al. (2009, p. 352, citing Rootman & Gordon-El-Bihbety, 2008) Wu et al. (2010, p. 444, citing Rootman & Gordon-El-Bihbety, 2008)	This definition is different from others in that it includes a communication component and specifies contexts. Unclear what is meant by or what constitutes *access, understand, evaluate, communicate information, promote, maintain, improve health* in adolescents. Unclear whose understanding is valued. Implies that a relationship exists between (a) accessing, understanding, evaluation, and communication of information and (b) the promotion, maintenance, and improvement of health in adolescents. The threshold at which health literacy is achieved in adolescents is not clear.
8	"health literacy is not limited to one's ability to **read** and **write**, but also encompasses **interactive and critical skills that resonate with a wellness and health promotion framework**." Massey et al. (2013, p. 342, citing Nutbeam, 2000)	Unclear what is meant by or what constitutes *read, write,* or *interactive and critical skills that resonate with a wellness and health promotion framework* in adolescents. The threshold at which health literacy is achieved in adolescents is not clear.
9	"In this paper, we use a definition of health literacy that focuses on each individual's capacity to **acquire** and **use new information**." Paek et al. (2011, p. 133, citing Baker, 2006)	Unclear what is meant by or what constitutes *acquire, use new information* in adolescents. The threshold at which health literacy is achieved in adolescents is not clear.
10	"health literacy (**understanding basic health terms**, ability to **follow medical instructions**)." Skopelja et al. (2008, p. 107, citing Norman & Skinner, 2006)	Unclear what is meant by or what constitutes *understanding basic health terms, follow medical instructions* in adolescents. Unclear whose understanding is valued. The threshold at which health literacy is achieved in adolescents is not clear.
11	"In its simplest form, health literacy is the ability to **understand** and **follow health instructions**." Wu et al. (2010, p. 445)	Unclear what is meant by or what constitutes *understand, follow health instructions* in adolescents. Unclear whose understanding is valued. The threshold at which health literacy is achieved in adolescents is not clear.
12	"health literacy occurs when the **skills** and **ability** of **those requiring health information and services** are aligned with the demand and complexity of **information and services**." Massey et al. (2013, p. 342, citing Ratzan & Parker, 2010)	Definition is different from others in that it specifies that health literacy occurs when a specific condition is met. Unclear who decides when the skills and ability of adolescents requiring health information and services are aligned with the demand and complexity of information and services. The skills and abilities of adolescents requiring health information and services are not specified.

Appendix. (Continued)

Row	Definitions and their source*	Analytical comments
13	"a health-literate person is able to **use health concepts and information generatively, applying information to novel situations**." Paek et al. (2011, p. 133, citing Zarcadoolas et al., 2006)	Definition is different from others in that it explicitly states conditions that must be met for an adolescent to be health literate. Unclear what is meant by or what constitutes *use, health concepts and information, generatively, applying, information, novel situations* in adolescents.
14	"Health literate individuals are able to **understand** and **apply health information** in **ways that allow them to take more control over their health** through, for example, appraising the credibility, accuracy and relevance of information and acting on that information to change their health behaviours or living conditions." Wu et al. (2010, p. 445)	Definition is different in that it specifies the condition in which adolescents are health literate. Unclear what is meant by or what constitutes *understand, apply,* or *health information*. Unclear whose understanding is valued. Unclear if all of the ways that adolescents can take control over their health are specified. Implies that a relationship exists between (a) understanding and applying health information and (b) adolescents taking more control over their health.
15	"health literacy is more than simply being able to **read pamphlets** and **make medical appointments**. It is basic literacy combined with **more advanced cognitive and social skills**, which empower people to be confident in their ability to **find, critique** and **process health information**." Paek et al. (2011, p. 133, citing Nutbeam, 2000)	Unclear what is meant by or what constitutes *basic literacy, more advanced social and cognitive skills, find, critique, process health information*. Implies that a relationship exists between (a) basic literacy, more advanced cognitive and social skills and (b) empowerment and confidence in adolescents' ability to find, critique, and process health information. The threshold at which health literacy is achieved in adolescents is not clear.

* Words in the definition that are vague or ambiguous are in bold font; words that are underlined have been modified by the author.

References

Berkman, N. D., Davis, T. C., & McCormack, L. (2010). Health literacy: What is it? *Journal of Health Communication, 15*(Suppl. 2), 9–19.

Brown, St. L., Teufel, J. A., Birch, D. A. (2007). Early adolescents' perceptions of health and health literacy. *Journal of School Health, 77*(1), 7–15.

Chang, L-C. (2011). Health literacy, self-reported status and health promoting behaviours for adolescents in Taiwan. *Journal of Clinical Nursing, 20*(1–2), 190–196.

Diamond, C., Saintonge, S., August, P., & Azrack, A. (2011). The development of Building Wellness™, a youth health literacy program. *Journal of Health Communication, 16*(Suppl. 3), 103–118.

Ghaddar, S. F., Valerio, M. A., Garcia, C. M., & Hansen, L. (2012). Adolescent health literacy: The importance of credible sources of online health information. *Journal of School Health, 82*(1), 28–36.

Gray, N. J., Klein, J. D., Noyce, P. R., Sesselberg, T. S., & Cantrill, J. A. (2005). The internet: A window on adolescent health literacy. *Journal of Adolescent Health, 37*(3), 243.c1–c7.

Hughes, W. (1996). *Critical thinking*. Peterborough, ON: Broadview Press.

Massey, P., Prelip, M., Calimlim, B., Afifi, A., Quiter, E., Nessim, S. ... Glik, D. (2013). Findings toward a multidimensional measure of adolescent health literacy. *American Journal of Health Behavior, 37*(3), 342–350.

Miles, M. B., & Huberman, A. M. (1994). *Qualitative data analysis: An expanded sourcebook* (2nd ed.). Thousand Oaks, CA: SAGE.

Paek, H., Reber, B. H., & Lariscy, R. W. (2011). Roles of interpersonal and media socialization agents in adolescent self-reported health literacy: A health socialization perspective. *Health Education Research, 26*(1), 131–149.

Peerson, A., & Saunders, M. (2009). Health literacy revisited: What do we mean and why does it matter? *Health Promotion International, 24*(3), 285–296.

Peterson, F. L., Cooper, R. J., & Laird, J. M. (2001). Enhancing teacher health literacy in school health promotion: A vision for the new millennium. *Journal of School Health, 71*(4), 138–144.

Petticrew, M., & Roberts, H. (2006). *Systematic reviews in the social sciences: A practical guide*. Malden, MA: Blackwell.

Ratzan, S. C., & Parker, R. M. (2000). Introduction. In C. R. Selden, M. Zorn, & R. M. Ratzan (Eds.), *National library of medicine current bibliographies in medicine: Health literacy* (pp. v–vi; NLM Pub. No. CMB 2000-1). Bethesda, MD: National Institutes of Health, U.S. Department of Health and Human Services.

Rootman, I., & Gordon-El-Bihbety, D. (2008). *A vision for a health literate Canada: Report of the expert panel on health literacy*. Ottawa, ON: Canadian Public Health Association. Retrieved from http://www.cpha.ca/ uploads/portals/h-l/report_e.pdf.

Rudd, R. E., McCray, A. T., & Nutbeam, D. (2012). Health literacy and definition of terms. In D. Begoray, D. Gillis, & G. Rowlands (Eds.), *Health literacy in context* (pp. 13–32). Hauppage, NY: Nova Science.

Sanders, L. M., Shaw, J. S., Guez, G., Baur, C., & Rudd, R. E. (2009). Health literacy and child health promotion: Implications for research, clinical care, and public policy. *Pediatrics, 124*(Suppl. 3), S306–S314.

Skopelja, E. N., Whipple, E. C., & Richwine, P. (2008). Reaching and teaching teens: Adolescent health literacy and the Internet. *Journal of Consumer Health on the Internet, 12*(2), 105–118.

Sorensen, K., Van den Broucke, S., Fullam, J., Doyle, G., Pelikan, J., Slonska, Z. ... HLS-EU Consortium. (2012). Health literacy and public health: A systematic review and integration of definitions and models. *BMC Public Health, 12*(80). doi:10.1186/1471-2458-12-80.

Vardavas, C. I., Kondilis, B. K., Patelarou, E., Akrivos, P. D., & Falagas, M. E. (2009). Health literacy and sources of health education among adolescents in Greece. *International Journal of Adolescent Medicine & Health, 21*(2), 179–186.

Wharf Higgins, J., Begoray, D., & MacDonald, M. (2009). A sociological conceptual framework for understanding adolescent health literacy in the health education classroom. *American Journal of Community Psychology, 44*(3–4), 350–362.

World Health Organization. (2015). *Adolescent development.* Geneva, Switzerland: Author. Retrieved from http://www.who.int/maternal_ child_adolescent/topics/adolescence/dev/en/

Wu, A. D., Begoray, D., MacDonald, M., Wharf Higgins, J. Frankish, J., Kwan, B. … Rootman, I. (2010). Developing and evaluating a relevant and feasible instrument for measuring health literacy of Canadian high school students. *Health Promotion International, 25*(4), 444–452.

In: Adolescent Health Literacy and Learning
Editors: D. L. Begoray and E. M. Banister
ISBN: 978-1-63482-897-0

Chapter 3

READING *CHASING ADLAND*: MIDDLE YEARS' STUDENTS IN PURSUIT OF CRITICAL MEDIA HEALTH LITERACY

Deborah Begoray* and Hong Fu
Department of Curriculum and Instruction, University of Victoria, Canada

ABSTRACT

The purpose of this study was to explore the responses of middle years' students to the graphic novel *Chasing Adland*. We observed lessons then conducted and transcribed interviews with students and teacher participants. Data analysis revealed several themes. Students focused on the nature of false reality in advertising and made personal connections. The teacher was impressed by the usefulness of the graphic novel and its concepts as part of an advertising unit. Both students and the teacher commented on critical media health literacy, advertising targeting as a gender issue, and the graphic novel as an enjoyable resource. We concluded that *Chasing Adland* is an effective addition to health literacy learning in the middle years' classroom.

Keywords: graphic novel, critical media health literacy, middle years

INTRODUCTION

Focusing Questions

1. Why are adolescents targeted by the commercial media?
2. What is the role of critical thinking in health literacy for adolescents?

The health literacy of adolescents is of particular importance in modern Canadian society. Knowing how to "access, understand, evaluate, and communicate information as a way to

* Correspondence to (email): dbegoray@uvic.ca

promote, maintain, and improve health in a variety of settings" (Rootman & Gordon-El-Bihbety, 2008, p. 3) is a prerequisite to health (Hoffman-Goetz, Donelle, & Ahmed, 2014) across the life course. In addition, there is a notably strong correspondence between health and health behaviours in adolescence and a continuation of these patterns in adulthood (Viner et al., 2012).

There is specific and aggressive targeting of adolescents by the commercial media, especially by the tobacco (Anderson, 2011; Minaker, Ahmed, Hammond, & Manske, 2014), alcohol (Weintraub Austin & Hust, 2005), food and beverage (Palmer & Carpenter, 2006; Weber, Story, & Harnack, 2006), and fashion industries (Isaksen & Roper, 2012). Adolescents report high levels of interaction with a variety of media (Rideout, Foehr, & Roberts, 2010). Some of this interaction is with sites that engage them with positive health messages (e.g., government public health information). The influence of the commercial media, however, affects not only their physical health but also their feelings of self-worth or what makes them feel healthy and well among their peers (Isaksen & Roper, 2012). It is, therefore, important that media influences on health/wellness — for better or worse — be part of the learning at school, one of the few institutions that touches the lives of almost all adolescents.

School health curricula are informed by research. There is, however, a lack of research on adolescent health compared to studies focused on children and adults. Scholars have called for more investigations on adolescent health (Manganello, 2008; Diamond, Saintonge, August, & Azrack, 2011); our research helps to address that call. Teachers, however, need resources based on research. For this reason, we developed a dissemination project employing the creation of a graphic novel suitable for use in a health education class.

Chasing Adland (Tran-Nguyen, Van Acken, Haberlin, Coe, & Dunn-Krahn, 2013) is a graphic novel that features a storyline with adolescent-aged characters and integrates messages about critical literacy, advertising, health literacy, and media literacy. *Chasing Adland* was written by adolescents for an audience of adolescents and professionally illustrated by an adult artist. It arose from a request by a middle years' teacher, Mrs. Day (all study participant names are pseudonyms), who wanted reading/viewing material for her students that would serve as a touchstone text to teach a unit on literacy, media, and health education. Mrs. Day had been a participant in previous phases of our multipart, mixed-methods research project (Begoray, Banister, Wharf Higgins, & Wilmot, 2015; Begoray, Wharf Higgins, Harrison, & Collins-Emery, 2013; Begoray, Wharf Higgins, & MacDonald, 2009; Begoray, Wharf Higgins, & Wilmot, 2014) and was eager to participate in another qualitative study.

BACKGROUND

Our research team has primarily adopted a *social determinants of health* (World Health Organization, 2011) approach to our research. We do, however, acknowledge both the biological and social influences on health behaviours in adolescence, which is "the key period for the adoption of health behaviours relating to substance misuse, sex, diet and exercise, and the self-management of chronic disorders" (Viner et al., 2012, p. 1648). Adolescents' physical, social, and emotional development and their cognitive skills are in a state of rapid change. They become more able to engage in abstract thinking and reasoning. At the same time, they have more autonomy and make more health decisions for themselves. As Manganello (2008) noted "[t]hese changes make adolescence an appropriate time to begin thinking about health literacy interventions" (p. 841).

The media are a major influence on adolescent health. In fact, the Centre for Media and Child Health says the media are "an environmental health issue" (Rich, 2013, p. 456); and we maintain that any significant intervention into adolescent health must take into account the pervasiveness of the media. In previous work, we have theorized that an individual's health literacy exists in a web of relationships or in a social ecology (Wharf Higgins, Begoray, & MacDonald, 2009) that includes family, peers, governments, and the media. These more proximal and more distal influences can be passively or actively encountered by individuals. It is our hope that giving adolescents the ability to evaluate messages they receive from all sources, but especially from the media, will allow them to take charge of their own health decisions.

"[H]ealth literacy skills (which include media literacy and critical thinking) are necessary for adolescents to be able to access health information from mass media, understand the content and evaluate the credibility of the information they obtain" (Manganello, 2008, p. 847). The use of media can promote healthy behaviours or can lead adolescents to more risk. This project sought to engage students in the development of a questioning stance, rather than merely seeking to inoculate them against media messages. In our previous work, we have noted that adolescents in health education classes can learn to make independent decisions and position themselves to accept or reject media messages (Begoray et al., 2012); we maintain that this is an important subset of health literacy, which we have termed *critical media health literacy* (Wharf Higgins & Begoray, 2012).

The schools are one important site for the development of critical media health literacy. All health literacy education is interdisciplinary; it is influenced by health education and literacy education. British Columbia's (BC) newly revised English Language Arts curriculum document (BC Ministry of Education [MOE], 2013a) stipulates that how adolescents "acquire knowledge and communicate" is rapidly changing, particularly with the advent of a more "digital environment" and that, therefore "[s]tudents must be able to critically evaluate and use multiple sources of information" (n.p.). This development of critical thinking, which becomes easier for students after puberty, can "involve students in asking questions about language and power and help them to read and rewrite the texts, narratives, and discourses that shape their lives, opportunities and the larger social order" (Ashcraft, 2012, p. 600). The BC English Language Arts Grade 7 curriculum (MOE, 2013a), for example, lists as a learning standard that students need to "think critically about the accuracy, reliability, and relevance of information" (n.p.); and a learning standard of the Grade 7 Physical and Health Education curriculum (MOE, 2013b) states that students should be able to access and evaluation health information, and understand "factors that influence personal health decisions, including the media and peers" (n.p.).

Thus, we have theorized a concept that looks at the overlap of skills in critical literacy, media literacy, and health literacy: critical media health literacy. We define critical media health literacy (CMHL) "as a right of citizenship and empowers individuals and groups, in a risky consumer society, to critically interpret and use media as a means to engage in decision-making processes and dialogues; exert control over their health and everyday events; and make healthy changes for themselves and their communities" (Wharf Higgins & Begoray,

2012, p. 142). We include adolescents as well as adults as those who have this *right of citizenship* and have endeavoured in our own research to assist teachers to engage students in discussions and activities that promote CMHL as part of making personal health decisions.

Specifically for adolescents, our own previous research and the professional literature in this area indicate that there are four main concepts that students need to understand to be critically media health literate:

Concept 1. Advertisements are ubiquitous, aggressive, and intent on controlling the purchasing habits of adolescents to benefit corporations. Students learn to ask: What does this ad want me to do?

Concept 2. Advertisements often create false reflections of reality particularly related to health, beauty, fitness, and happiness. Students learn to ask: Is this depiction realistic? Does it match with my understanding of the world around me?

Concept 3. Advertisements attract adolescents using *hooks*. Students learn to ask: What is this ad promising in order to attract my attention? How is this advertisement trying to catch my attention?

Concept 4. Adolescents can learn to recognize and then accept or reject media-perpetuated identities and values. Students learn to ask: What kind of person does this ad want me to be? Do I want to be that person? What values does this advertisement promote? Do I share those values?

The school has become responsible in many jurisdictions for not just the traditional school subjects (e.g., English and mathematics) but to address society's larger issues such as the impact of technology. MediaSmarts (2014), a Canadian not-for-profit charitable organization, commented that "schools are an important source of digital literacy education, with almost half of students relying on teachers to learn about online issues" (para. 2) including advertising. Health education leading to greater health literacy needs to include attention to advertising messages that pertain to health.

Media, of course, come in many guises: social media such as Facebook™, Twitter™; web sites; more traditional mass media such as newspapers, magazines, and television. As noted above, any of these formats can be used positively or negatively for health education. We decided to use yet another media format, the comic book style graphic novel, as a main feature of our research. The creation of *Chasing Adland* and its use in Mrs. Day's classroom led to a further research opportunity on the responses of the teacher and students to this resource.

DESCRIPTION OF THE *CHASING ADLAND* WRITING PROJECT

Graphic Novel

A graphic novel is a book-length, fiction or nonfiction story produced in the style of a comic book (Danzak, 2011). The use of a graphic novel created by adolescent students was the focus of the study described in this chapter. It is 24 pages in length; each page is one-half of an 8.5×11.0 inch sheet of paper that has a number of panels — as many as four and as few as one. While shorter than many graphic novels, its length did not seem to detract from its classroom usefulness or from its appeal for our study's adolescent readers, many of whom were avid graphic novel enthusiasts in their out-of-school lives. The growing popularity of the graphic novel as a genre that connects life and school provides teachers with a useful pedagogical tool for media literacies (Schwarz & Crenshaw, 2011). In fact the teacher, Mrs. Day, who piloted the novel, valued it as an appealing, illustrated narrative that could be quickly read and viewed by students and yet still provide an abundance of ideas for CMHL lessons. Research shows, however, that 'reading' graphica of all types needs instruction so students more fully understand the visual messages (Pantaleo, 2014). We provided assistance to Mrs. Day in the form of ideas for addressing visual messages.

Writers and Workshop Process

As research fellows of the Centre for Youth and Society at the University of Victoria (http://www.youth.society.uvic.ca/), we had seen a graphic novel completed by a group of incarcerated youth that addressed the issue of the high rate of return to prison by youth breaking their probation. When we received the request for graphic novel reading material from Mrs. Day, we decided to create a similar product that would involve embedding principles of this different context within a narrative framework. Our opportunity came in the summer of 2012 when the Greater Victoria Public Library agreed to add a graphic novel writing workshop to their summer course offerings for adolescents if we would offer it free of charge. Five students, aged 13 and 14 years, attended.

Facilitated by a graduate student research assistant who is also an experienced teacher and by an adult photographer/youth worker, the students spent 15 hours (3 hours per day for a week) learning about CMHL, writing the story, creating storyboards, and posing for panels to create their graphic novel. Posed panels were photographed, and these pictures became the basis for the adult illustrator to create the finished graphic novel. The student writers called their finished comic *Chasing Adland* (Tran-Nguyen et al., 2013).

Chasing Adland: Plot Summary

The adolescent writers created a storyline they thought would be engaging for other adolescents. The main character, Chase, is teased by other girls about her clothes and becomes convinced that a new wardrobe will change her life. Her mother declines to finance a shopping trip. Adman appears to Chase in a dream and lures her to Adland, a mall with everything that Chase wants and where things seem to be free. There she meets Celebrity Girl, who also urges her to buy, and Luke, a boy who joins Chase in her shopping spree. However, Chase's curiosity about a trapdoor in the mall introduces them to a darker land. A more realistic looking, less photo-shopped version of Celebrity Girl tells them they have entered Real Adland, where there are grim factories and imitation products designed for commercials. Chase awakes from her dream determined to be herself and on her way to school rejects the comments of other girls on her clothes. Chase then meets Luke who wants to be her friend. As the novel ends, we see Adman luring Chase's tormentors to the mall.

The Study: Reading *Chasing Adland*

We asked the question: What is the response of a teacher and a class of middle years' students to a graphic novel containing concepts of critical media health literacy as they pertain to advertising? The research took place over a 3-week period in April 2014. Mrs. Day engaged her Grades 7 and 8 students with *Chasing Adland* for six lessons, each of which lasted from 25 to 60 minutes. During the last two lessons, two student teachers participated by working individually with students for some activities.

METHOD

Setting

The research setting was a middle school in a lower socioeconomic suburban area in a mid-sized city on Canada's west coast. Our work was designed in part "to bridge the gap between university-based theorists and school based practitioners in a way that treated teachers as knowledge producers" (Corbett, 2010, p. 668). This study was no exception with Mrs. Day taking a major role as planner, instructor, observer, and informant.

Participants

At the time of the research project, students ranged in age from 12–14 years. The teacher described the class as "average kids" who were "not terribly diverse in their abilities." Of the 15 students in this classroom, 10 participated in the research project; five girls and five boys; six were in Grade 7 and four were in Grade 8; one boy, Jeff, was Aboriginal (see Table 1). Students and their parent/guardian signed letters of informed consent. The research study was approved by the University of Victoria Human Research Ethics Board.

Table 1. Study Participants

Name (pseudonyms)	M/F	Grade	Age
Kate	F	7	12
Missy	F	7	12
Alice	F	7	13
Vanessa	F	7	12
Debi	F	7	12
Sheldon	M	8	13
John	M	8	14
Tim	M	7	13
Norm	M	8	14
Jeff	M	8	14

Mrs. Day had 20 years of experience in the classroom and held a masters' degree in literacy education. While she had made good use of advertisements from magazines and

YouTube™ as classroom resources in the past, she wanted reading material to anchor a unit on media literacy that focused on advertising.

Before this study began, we provided Mrs. Day with materials that contained ideas for teaching *Chasing Adland* prepared by two members of the research team who both had extensive experience teaching in the middle years' classroom. A major component in these materials was an article (Begoray, Wharf Higgins, & Wilmot, 2014) with activities designed to help achieve learning standards from the BC English Language Arts (MOE, 2013a), Social Studies (MOE, 2013b), and Physical and Health Education (MOE, 2013c) curricula. Mrs. Day, like many middle years' teachers, uses an interdisciplinary instructional approach incorporating outcomes from a number of different subjects in a single lesson. These lessons were no exception.

Data Collection

Observations of Six Lessons

Yin (2009) noted that "observations of the ... curriculum at work are valuable aids for understanding the actual uses of the curriculum" (p. 110). A graduate student research assistant attended every class and took notes on the lesson procedures. These observations were corroborated by a second observer at every lesson. All notes were transcribed for analysis.

Interviews

Semi-structured individual interviews took place with Mrs. Day and all 10 students. We used interviews in order to seek the insights of the teacher and the students so as to understand in part their "perceived causal inferences and explanations" (Yin, 2009, p. 110) of their response to the graphic novel. Mrs. Day was interviewed for 40 minutes during lunch hour in a private room by a member of the research team (see Appendix A for teacher interview questions). The students were interviewed during lunch hour for 10–20 minutes in the private room by one of two members of the research team (see Appendix B for student interview questions).

Data Analysis

Transcripts were examined for salient themes and categories during a semantic analysis (Cohen & Manion, 1992; Patton, 2002). Categories were refined as analysis continued (Glaser & Strauss, 1967; Huberman & Miles, 1994). The approach used to process the data was analytic induction (Goetz & LeCompte, 1981), which enabled researchers to "explore the data without prior hypotheses" (Best & Kahn, 1993, p. 186) and, therefore, allow meaning to emerge from the data (Hood, 2007). Written observations and recorded interviews were transcribed by a member of the research team and then analyzed by another research team member. The coding process followed an approach described as lean coding (Creswell, 2014), which uses hand coding to determine initial codes, categories, and themes as well as to identify important participant quotations.

Overview of the Six Lessons

Lesson 1

The first lesson started with a brief assessment of students' prior knowledge of media and media literacy (Gainer, 2010). Mrs. Day introduced the four concepts of CMHL (described earlier) by posting them on the wall; these posted concepts were frequently referred to in later sessions. The students placed sticky notes on a concept poster to indicate their familiarity with a particular concept. Of the four, only Concept 3 had any sticky notes attached showing that students believed they understood only that: advertisements attract adolescents using hooks. After that, the class viewed the cover page of the book (Figure 1) projected on a screen and offered their predictions about the book's plot and characters.

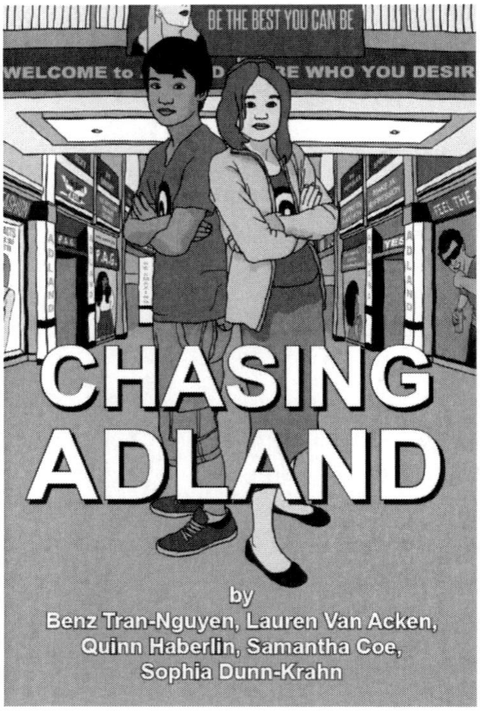

Figure 1. Cover page of *Chasing Adland* (Tran-Nguyen et al., 2013).

Lesson 2

Mrs. Day began by informing students that the authors of *Chasing Adland* were also middle years' students. She projected the images from the first pages with the print blacked out and directed students to observe the images carefully, then discuss the characters and setting, and finally predict what would happen next. She targeted Concepts 1 and 2 in particular by posing questions such as "Who benefits from ads?" and "What do ads want you to do?" Students responded to the questions in pairs.

Lesson 3

In a whole-class discussion, students continued to actively read the images first and tried to get as much information as possible from the images as well as the print text. They offered their views on the character of Adman and the Adland Mall, and Mrs. Day provided her interpretation of the visual symbols depicted in the book (such as the bulls' eye on Chase's and Luke's t-shirts). The lesson ended with Mrs. Day asking students to pose a question about CMHL as a 'ticket out the door'; that is, they were instructed to tell her their question before being allowed to leave the classroom for lunch.

Lesson 4

Mrs. Day began by asking questions designed to relate CMHL to the students' experiences with advertising. They continued to read/view the book and make predictions about what else might happen during Chase's and Luke's experiences in Adland Mall. The whole-class discussion branched off to other topics as determined by student interest, such as celebrity and fandom. Finally, Mrs. Day directed the discussion back to Concepts 1, 2, and 3 and encouraged students to discuss how these concepts were reflected in the book.

Lesson 5

Mrs. Day asked students to fill in a two-column sheet to summarize their knowledge of CMHL and to compare notes with each other. They continued to read/view the remaining part of the book. The whole-class discussion that followed branched off to areas that interested the class, such as how advertisers sometimes seek to fool consumers. While critically reading the book, students posed questions such as who Adman was working for. The lesson ended with a discussion on the trap door leading to Real Adland that Chase was eager to open while Luke was reluctant. Students compared the reactions and speculated on the characters' reasons.

Lesson 6

In the final lesson, the class formed four table groups and acted as what Mrs. Day called "ad detectives" to find evidence of the four concepts in the book. They filled in a worksheet individually while engaging in small-group discussion. Then they compared notes by gossiping; that is, they employed a technique called GOSSIP (Go Out and Selectively Search for Important Points; Close, 2011). They moved about the room getting ideas from people in other groups and adding those ideas they found important to their own sheets. Mrs. Day then commented on the four concepts one by one, and the students summarized new knowledge about CMHL they had learnt from all the lessons.

FINDINGS

Observation Themes of Six Lessons

There were two observation themes of the six lessons: the use of the four CMHL concepts and the value of the graphic novel genre for teaching reading/viewing comprehension and evaluation.

Use of Four CMHL Concepts

Mrs. Day focused on the four concepts, or "big ideas" of CMHL as she referred to them in the teacher interview (see below), by introducing the concepts in the very first session, constantly referring back to them in the succeeding sessions, posting them on the bulletin board, and concluding the lesson sequence with them. She used them to focus lessons, as a source of questions, and as a structure for the lesson sequence.

Reading/Viewing Comprehension and Evaluation

Comic style books could easily be read quickly for just the plot. Mrs. Day, who stated in the interview that the ease of reading is one of the appeals of *Chasing Adland* (see below), nevertheless slowed down the process to encourage close reading of images as well as the print. Throughout the lessons, she encouraged students to access their prior knowledge by asking for student experiences with advertising and shopping. She also did extensive work with prediction exercises that involved students using prior knowledge about characters and stories to actively engage in speculating what future events in the story might be. For example, villains such as Adman are often defeated; would the same thing happen in this story?

The class worked individually, in pairs, in small groups, and as a whole class. Both the teacher and students contributed to the class discussions and raised questions concerning the book. The lessons were co-constructed with the teacher frequently leading, but students also engaged in social construction with one another in a process of dialogic inquiry (Reznitskaya, 2012): "In dialogic classrooms, teachers and students act as co-inquirers, collaboratively engaging in a generation and evaluation of new interpretations of texts in order to 'gain a fuller appreciation of the world, [them]selves, and one another'" (Burbules as cited in Reznitskaya, 2012, p. 446). For example, the students became interested in particular characters and settings in the book, posed questions, and stated their opinions about them; the teacher also shared her views with students; thus, the discussions provided a valuable opportunity for reading the book in multiple ways. Furthermore, Mrs. Day allowed students to lead the discussion away from the book's plot to other related topics, such as nature of celebrity, fandom, and logos. They also commented freely on the book itself as a construction, with debates over authors' intent, effectiveness of the story, and the skill of the illustrator.

With these intentional measures to facilitate understanding and promote reflection, the students learnt to tease out the subtle messages from the ads in the book and to critically examine them by asking questions such as "Who benefits?" and "What does this ad want me/teenagers to do?"

Student Interview Themes

Two main themes emerged in the student interviews: the recognition that advertisers take liberties with the concept of reality (i.e., consumers must remain alert to judge what is real and not real) and that one way adolescents can understand advertisements is to make personal connections with their own experiences.

Real and Not Real

Mrs. Day stated that a main part of teaching CMHL in this novel was to help students consider what is real and not real, and this topic emerged as a theme in student interviews. For example, several students identified the contrast of glamorous Adland Mall to Real Adland. This stark juxtaposition was frequently mentioned by students as the most interesting part of the novel. John, 14, Grade 8: "It's like you assumed everything was nice, like perfect and then you got the hard realization that this isn't always so nice, it's kind of a facade to what's actually going on." Alice, 13, Grade 7: "[This part] tells you what it's really like and that the other Adland [Mall] is just fake ... it tells people the actual truth." Sheldon, 13, Grade 8: "[This contrast] shows how people can get so overwhelmed with buying stuff and find out that it's really just fake." One student summarized by observing that the main message of the graphic novel seemed to be: "Watch out for … ads. Make sure that they don't lie to you." (Jeff, 14, Grade 8).

Personal Connections to Individual Experiences

Students made a variety of personal connections to events in *Chasing Adland.* For example, the alteration of Celebrity Girl's appearance in Real Adland prompted comments about photo-shopping. Missy (12, Grade 7) observed that models in ads are "photo shopped. I watched a video about it last year ... her leg was like this [gestures outwards in a curve] but they could cave it in so it would be skinny." She was also critical of advertisements in Adland Mall that seem to promise that contact lenses would make girls prettier. She offered another connection to her own life: "Contacts are way more complicated. I tried it for Halloween and it didn't work."

Another student, Tim (13, Grade 7), was interested in how health and well-being was implicated in advertising. While he offers his comment using second person 'you', it seems to address his own experience: "Some fashion could harm you in a way because of how angry some people get. They'll get jealous ... so next day you'll have, like, you have something really important in your locker and they somehow figured out your locker combination and got that thing." The teacher had encouraged personal connections in the lessons, and this behaviour continued in the interviews.

Teacher Interview Themes

Two main themes emerged from the interview with Mrs. Day. They included, first, the usefulness of *Chasing Adland* to teach an advertising unit and, second, the usefulness of the CMHL concepts as teaching tools.

Graphic Novel as Touchstone for the Unit

As noted above, it was Mrs. Day who first requested reading material to focus an advertising unit (done as part of a previous research project) that had been formerly based on viewing and discussing advertisements and creating advertisements: "That was the one thing that was missing when we did the first unit. There wasn't anything to … bring all the ideas together." During her interview she mused about how previous ideas and this graphic novel might work together in a larger unit. She speculated that she "would probably use it throughout the unit as a touchstone."

Usefulness of the Four Concepts

As we observed in the lessons (see above), Mrs. Day made full use of the four concepts. She returned to this theme in the interview as well. She noted that the BC curricula (MOE,

2013a, 2013b, 2013c) has moved toward an overall reduction in learning outcomes and has substituted a small number of what she terms "big ideas" that are a "framework to hang your hat on." The idea of four main ideas of CMHL was for her a familiar concept: "You can take those four concepts and frame them as the four big ideas." In addition, Mrs. Day described how she had noticed that her students had adopted and had begun to "use the language of the big ideas" and that she had overheard students connecting big ideas to events in the graphic novel. She reported one student saying to another "You're not being honest — remember in Adland," which she believed showed students referring to Concept 2, that is, advertisements often create false reflections of reality.

Themes Shared by Students and Teachers

Three common themes emerged in our analysis of the student and teacher interviews: discussing and understanding CMHL, debating the issue of whether advertising is primarily a girls' issue or problem, and finding enjoyment in the novel.

Understanding CMHL

When asked by interviewers, many of the students were able to define CMHL, offering definitions such as: "It means to read the ad, or look at the ad, and kind of process it yourself, and to critically think about the ad and what it's telling you, what it wants you to do. And you decide if you want to do that." (Kate, 12, Grade 7), and "I think it means to be aware of what the point of the ad is, and also to realize what the ads want me to do, what ads want me to think" (John, 14, Grade 8).

The students were generally able to engage critically with the concepts the novel introduced, speculating on motivation for advertisements, such as "People spend their money on, like, what's in, so that's why they don't make things last very long, so they'll buy their next new big product" (Vanessa, 12, Grade 7). They also grappled with the abstract idea that ads may be part of the fabric of our society. For example, Tim (13, Grade 7) states this conundrum: "I don't like advertising, [but] if we didn't have advertisements, we'd have a lot higher TV bill ... right?" perhaps referring to some countries such as the UK that charge viewers a television license.

Advertising Targeting As a Gender Issue

There was some evidence from Mrs. Day that boys see targeting by advertisers as a girls' issue. The novel features Chase as the female protagonist, but she meets Luke at Adland Mall. Luke also shops and is lured by ads with muscular male models. Mrs. Day commented: "I found it really interesting that both the boys and girls latched onto ... the advertising geared towards girls.... I had to draw them into the boy part … [but] they would always just talk about Celebrity Girl or the '95% prettier' [store sign]. I thought they would clue into the steroid guy [a photo in an ad in the novel] ... but they didn't."

While it was certainly true that students did not talk about the boy-focussed advertising in classroom lessons, the interviews revealed that some students did notice gender-based ads, though they differed in what they thought the difference might be, if any. For example, Kate (12, Grade 7) pointed out that "on page 2 [a sign says] 'New contacts. Be yourself. 95% prettier' and then on page 10 it says 'Be a Man.' So that is pretty much the same too, because not all people, guys, want to be a 'Man' and they don't want to work out and they just want to be themselves." Another girl tries to articulate what the difference might be between advertising directed at boys and that directed at girls: "[Luke] is trying to pick out something about sport so he'll be like ... more recognizable, and [Chase] is trying to like … pick out makeup and trying to look like Celebrity Girl that was photo shopped to look perfect" (Missy, 12, Grade 7).

Student Enjoyment

Chasing Adland, according to both teacher and students, was enjoyable. Mrs. Day commented that she noticed her students "really had a connection with Chase," the main protagonist. She also reported on classroom events that occurred outside of observed lessons on the novel. She was thrilled that her students had adopted the events of the novel as a shared classroom community experience: "Someone brought in something to eat and someone [else] said that it looked as good as something you would see in Adland. Like they are playing around with it. They're getting it!" Students themselves in interviews also identified the novel as enjoyable. One identified visuals as appealing: "I love [the book] ... 'cause a lot of the information came from the pictures" (Kate, 12, Grade 7). Another student wanted to share his enjoyment of the novel's satiric word play in advertisements: "[There's a store in the novel called] PAG! Pretty awesome.... There is actually a brand called GAP and PAG is GAP backwards!" (Tim, 13, Grade 7).

Discussion

"Ads and all that are defining kids' lives now." (Norm, 14, Grade 8). Findings seem to indicate that *Chasing Adland* was an enjoyable, age-appropriate resource to introduce middle years' students to the concepts of CMHL. Students responded to the characters, to Chase more so than Luke; to the setting of Adland Mall and the contrasting Real Adland; and understood the concepts of CMHL. They engaged in critical discussion, connected to personal experiences, and even adopted the discourse of the novel.

One important fact about *Chasing Adland* contributing to its success in this classroom may have been its authorship. Mrs. Day commented: "I love that it was made by kids. I think that my kids liked that it was done by kids. It was a good door opener because this isn't just something that adults are pushing." We noted also that Mrs. Day delivered lessons that engaged her students in authentic discussion, weaving in new ideas as she saw opportunities and giving students active roles in small groups and as individuals to further interact with the novel's concepts. Moreover, they began to play with its ideas and language. One of the big ideas for the new draft English Language Arts curriculum is that "Language and literature help us find meaning and joy" (MOE, 2013a, n.p.). We see evidence of students finding both in these lessons.

Ultimately however, we were interested in the responses of these adolescents, their critical thinking about the commercial media; and these students were forthcoming when we asked about their questions. John (14, Grade 8) mused: "One question that came to mind ... Am I influenced by ads? Like, what if I don't even realize ... that it's kind of a subconscious thing ... like when they talk about how they do so much research on kids and I'm thinking like 'whoa, that's kind of scary how much they research just to put in an ad!'" As Celebrity Girl says to Chase in *Chasing Adland:* "We know you very well." Students in this classroom seemed to be able to understand and critically evaluate during and after the lessons.

LIMITATIONS

There were, of course, limitations to our study. One was the possibility of reflexivity (Yin, 2009) during both classroom observations and in the interviews. Yin cautioned that observed events may be influenced by being observed and that interviewees may give opinions based on what they believe interviewers want to hear. However, the influence on classroom lessons and the teacher interview may have been lessened by the teacher's familiarity with research team members since we had worked in her classroom before. Mrs. Day's students were less familiar with us, having only seen us as occasional classroom observers.

A second limitation is that we cannot establish cause and effect; that is, we do not know that students grew in CMHL. We did not ask in an interview or pretest what they knew about CMHL before reading *Chasing Adland.* However, our observation of the first lesson showed that, when presented with the four concepts of CMHL, the students perceived that they only understood one concept: advertising hooks. As described in Lesson 1, they indicated this belief by attaching sticky notes to the poster with the four concepts. Only Concept 3 (i.e., advertisements attract adolescents using hooks) had notes attached. Unfortunately, Mrs. Day did not repeat this same exercise in the final lesson so we have no direct comparison of whether or not they believed their understanding of the four concepts had advanced. We do, however, have the expert opinion of the teacher that the students did grow in their understanding of CMHL.

IMPLICATIONS FOR PRACTICE

A number of implications for teaching practice can be inferred from this study. Primarily designed as an instructional resource for the middle years' classroom, *Chasing Adland* seems to be both effective and engaging for the teaching of outcomes within English language arts and health education. Its graphic novel format provides both print and visual message systems to convey the four concepts of CMHL. Its narrative and characters are age appropriate, and events portrayed are common to urban teenagers' experiences. *Chasing Adland* provides a model for other middle years' students and their teachers who may want to create a novel (Mrs. Day's class embarked on just such a project after our research was complete) or other health education materials for their peers. The comic book format is familiar to and popular with students. Other graphic novels on other topics might be sought out by middle years' teachers to teach subject area content other than advertising. Clinical settings might use *Chasing Adland*; it could be made available in hard copy in waiting rooms or posted on web sites. The story offers openings for discussions with individual adolescents not only on advertising and consumerism but also about the nature of friendship, body image, and self-confidence. The teacher's dialogic approach might be adopted by healthcare professionals as a way to engage adolescents in discussing health issues. There were, however, less successful features of this novel. Mrs. Day was asked specifically: What aspects of the novel's format weren't really effective? She replied, "I think maybe for the guys." The role of Luke and advertising's role in influencing boys' purchases may need more emphasis, and certainly teachers or clinicians would need to seek additional materials to supplement discussions with boys. Finally, despite the use of *Chasing Adland* and the accompanying lessons, some students still struggled to bring a critical lens to advertising. When asked to define CMHL, Alice (13, Grade 7) said, "It depends on if I like the product that they're trying to sell." She did not seem to grasp the idea of advertisers seeking to influence her opinion but seemed to see ads as neutral sources of information.

Implications for Research

Adolescent health literacy remains under-researched, despite its importance for a healthy population now and in the future. As new curricula on health education are introduced, as is the case in BC, researchers have the opportunity to both suggest instructional strategies to teachers and to investigate the outcomes of these and other health education approaches.

The commercial media remain a dominant player in the health of adolescents. Researchers can look as well at the influence of health-promoting media other than the graphic novel for adolescents' health behaviours. Not only viewing and reading but also design and creation of media such as web sites and video games for an audience of their peers might be researched to investigate how adolescents' health literacy is influenced by such activities.

The creation of a graphic novel is an innovative knowledge dissemination tool. As we searched for a better way to reach an audience of adolescents about an adolescent health literacy issue, the popularity of the graphic novel with this age group made it an appealing choice. Researchers might investigate other genres as ways to disseminate research, particularly for adolescents. Boys might be interested in video games that embed health education findings, for example.

Finally, this study raised the question of whether adolescents, especially boys, view the targeting of advertisers as primarily a girls' or women's issue. As Mrs. Day wondered, "Do the guys just think that this is a woman's problem or a woman's issue? I don't know." Researchers might explore whether such attitudes exist and, if so, how they might be addressed.

Conclusion

The adolescents who participated in this study demonstrated many of the aspects of CMHL such as empowerment, critical interpretation, and using media (in this case, a graphic novel) "as a means to engage in decision making processes and dialogues" (Wharf Higgins &

Begoray, 2012, p. 142). As such, this health literacy intervention seemed to be successful in engaging students. *Chasing Adland* was a highly useful resource. It must be noted, however, that this novel was introduced in a socially constructed space between students, a highly educated and experienced teacher, and a team of researchers working together. Even in absentia, the student authors and illustrator contributed to the lessons. Critical media health literacy for adolescents, it seems, is a right of citizenship that might best be fostered in a social ecological setting with all players interacting together.

Questions for Discussion, Reflection, and Writing

4. Which of the findings did you find most surprising? Least surprising?
5. What other health literacy topics might lend themselves to the creation of comic book style graphic novel by adolescents? Why do you think so?
6. Download *Chasing Adland* (http://www.gvpl.ca/assets/PDF/ Audiences/Teens/ Chasing-Adland.pdf) and read it for yourself. How might you use it with adolescents to teach health literacy?

List of Online Resources

- Media Smarts: Canada's Centre for Digital and Media Literacy – http://www. mediasmarts.ca
- National Association for Media Literacy Education – http://www.namle.net
- Cooperative Children's Book Center, School of Education, University of Wisconsin-Madison – http://ccbc.education.wisc.edu/books/ graphicnovels.asp
- Get Graphic – http://www.getgraphic.org/teachers.php

Appendix A. Interview Questions for the Teacher

1. *Chasing Adland* was designed as a teaching tool for educators discussing Critical Media Health Literacy (CMHL) with 11- and 12-year-old students. Could you briefly describe who you teach, your understanding of CMHL, and the way you approached this topic with your class.
2. Did you use the novel in conjunction with a larger curriculum that aimed to develop CMHL? If so, describe this process.
3. Describe how you used *Chasing Adland* in your overall CMHL unit? For example:
   - Was the novel used as an introduction, mid-unit, or at the end of the unit? Why? How effective was your placement of the novel?
   - Given that media-perpetuated messages are delivered largely through visuals, how effective was presenting CMHL concepts through graphic novel visuals?
   - Describe other ways that you used the novel to increase students' awareness of CMHL.

4. *Chasing Adland* was designed to provide visual and written prompts to stimulate discussion around CMHL key concepts. What aspects of the novel were particularly effective as a CMHL teaching tool? Why?
5. What aspects of the novel's format were not effective as a CMHL teaching tool? Why?
6. Do you have any other comments or suggestions for us as to the use of this graphic novel as a CMHL teaching tool?

APPENDIX B. INTERVIEW QUESTIONS FOR STUDENTS

1. I understand that you have been talking about how to critically read health messages that are delivered through the media in ads. Can you describe what you have been discussing in class? What does it mean to you to be *critically media health literate*?
2. Your teacher used a novel called *Chasing Adland* in the unit on media health messages. Thinking about health messages that are delivered through the media, what parts of the book did you find most interesting or meaningful to you as an adolescent? Why? (Provide students with copies of the novel to remind them of the story and to stimulate thought.)
3. We hoped that the visuals and the written story would give students the opportunity to discuss ways that the media affects health attitudes and behaviours and how adolescents can take charge of their own health by viewing media messages critically. What questions or thoughts came to mind as you viewed the novel's visuals and read the story?
4. How did this novel help you learn about what it means to view media health messages critically?
5. Were there parts of the book that were not effective as a CMHL teaching tool? Why?
6. Are there any suggestions that you have for us about the graphic novel?
7. Do you have any other comments about being a CMH-literate adolescent that would help us when talking with other adolescents?

REFERENCES

Anderson, S. J. (2011). Marketing of menthol cigarettes and consumer perceptions: A review of tobacco industry documents. *Tobacco Control, 20*(Suppl. 2), ii20–ii28. doi:10.1136/tc.2010.041939

Ashcraft, C. (2012). But how do we talk about it? Critical literacy practices for addressing sexuality with youth. *Curriculum Inquiry, 42*(5), 597–628.

Begoray, D., Banister, E., Wharf Higgins, J., & Wilmot, R. (2015). Puppets on a string? How young adolescents explore gender and health in advertising. *Journal of Media Literacy Education, 6*(3), 57–64.

Begoray, D., Wharf Higgins, J., Harrison, J., & Collins-Emery, A. (2013). Adolescent reading/viewing of advertisements: Understandings from transactional and positioning theory. *Journal of Adolescent & Adult Literacy, 57*(2), 121–130.

Begoray, D., Wharf Higgins, J., & MacDonald, M. (2009). High school health curriculum and health literacy: Canadian student voices. *Global Health Promotion, 16*(4), 35–42.

Begoray, D., Wharf Higgins, J., & Wilmot, R. (2014). *Chasing Adland*: Teaching critical media health literacy. *English Practice, 56*(1), 55–61.

Best, J. W., & Kahn, J. V. (1993). *Research in education* (7th ed.). Boston, MA: Allyn & Bacon.

British Columbia Ministry of Education. (2013a). *English language arts, grade 7*. Victoria, BC: Author. Retrieved from https://curriculum.gov.bc.ca/curriculum/English%20Language%20Arts/7

British Columbia Ministry of Education. (2013b). *Physical and health education, grade 7*. Victoria, BC: Author. Retrieved from https://curriculum.gov.bc.ca/curriculum/Physical%20and%20Health%20Education/7

British Columbia Ministry of Education. (2013c). *Social studies, grade 7*. Victoria, BC: Author. Retrieved from https://curriculum.gov.bc.ca/curriculum/Social%20Studies/7

Close, S. (2011). *BrainSmart tools: Powerful pathways for personalizing 21st century learning*. Vancouver, BC: Susan Close Learning. Retrieved from http://www.smartreading.ca/pdfs/brainsmart_tools_sept72012.pdf

Cohen, L., & Manion, L. (1992). *Research methods in education* (4th ed.). New York, NY: Routledge.

Corbett, M. (2010). Pedagogy as case study. In A. Mills, C. Durepos, & E. Wiebe (Eds.), *Encyclopedia of case study research* (pp. 665–671). Thousand Oaks, CA: SAGE.

Creswell, J. W. (2014). *Research design: Qualitative, quantitative, and mixed methods approaches* (4th ed.). Thousand Oaks, CA: SAGE.

Danzak, R. L. (2011). Defining identities through multiliteracies: EL teens narrate their immigration experiences as graphic stories. *Journal of Adolescent & Adult Literacy, 55*(3), 186–196.

Diamond, C., Saintonge, S., August, P., & Azrack, A. (2011). The development of Building Wellness™, a youth health literacy program. *Journal of Health Communication, 16*(Supp. 3), 103–118.

Gainer, J. (2010). Critical media literacy in middle school: Exploring the politics of representation. *Journal of Adolescent & Adult Literacy, 53*(5), 364–373.

Glaser, B., & Strauss, A. L. (1967). *The discovery of grounded theory: Strategies for qualitative research*. Hawthorne, NY: Aldine de Gryter.

Goetz, J. P., & LeCompte, M. D. (1981). Ethnographic research and the problem of data reduction. *Anthropology and Education Quarterly, 11*, 51–70.

Hoffman-Goetz, L., Donelle, L., & Ahmed, R. (2014). *Health literacy in Canada: A primer for students*. Toronto, ON: Canadian Scholars' Press.

Hood, J. (2007). Orthodoxy vs. power: The defining traits of grounded theory. In A. Bryant & K. Charmaz (Eds.), *The SAGE handbook of grounded theory* (pp. 151–164). Thousand Oaks, CA: SAGE.

Huberman, A. M., & Miles, M. B. (1994). Data management and analysis methods. In N. K. Denzin & Y. S. Lincoln (Eds.), *Handbook of qualitative research* (pp. 428–444): Thousand Oaks, CA: SAGE.

Isaksen, K. J., & Roper, S. (2012). The commodification of self-esteem: Branding and British teenagers. *Psychology & Marketing, 29*(3), 117–135.

Manganello, J. A. (2008). Health literacy and adolescents: A framework and agenda for future research. *Health Education Research, 23*(5), 840–847.

MediaSmarts. (2014). *Saskatchewan Government committed to teaching students to be safe and ethical online* [Press release]. Retrieved from http://us2.campaign-archive1.com/?u=67f408dfb22f2784ff7891486&id=42c523e08c&e=667834928d

Minaker, L. M, Ahmed, R., Hammond, D., & Manske, S. (2014). Flavored tobacco use among Canadian students in grades 9 through 12: Prevalence and patterns from the 2010–2011 youth smoking survey. *Preventing Chronic Disease: Public Health Research, Practice, and Policy, 11*, 140094. doi:http://dx.doi.org/10.5888/pcd11.140094

Palmer, E., & Carpenter, C. (2006). Food and beverage marketing to children and youth: Trends and issues. *Media Psychology, 8*(2), 165–190.

Pantaleo, S. (2014). Exploring the artwork in picturebooks with middle years' students. *Journal of Children's Literature, 40*(1), 15–26.

Patton, M. Q. (2002). *Qualitative research and evaluation methods* (3rd ed.). Thousand Oaks, CA: SAGE.

Reznitskaya, A. (2012). Dialogic teaching: Rethinking language use during literature discussions. *The Reading Teacher, 65*(7), 446–456.

Rich, M. (2013). The medical community in the U.S.: Treating media as an influence on health and development. In D. Lemish (Ed.), *The Routledge handbook of children, adolescents and the media* (pp. 451–458). New York, NY: Routledge.

Rideout, V. J., Foehr, U. G., & Roberts, D. F. (2010). *Generation M^2: Media in the lives of 8– to 18-year-olds.* Menlo Park, CA: Henry J. Kaiser Family Foundation. Retrieved from https://kaiserfamilyfoundation.files. wordpress.com/2013/04/8010.pdf

Rootman, I., & Gordon-El-Bihbety, D. (2008). *A vision for a health literate Canada: Report of the expert panel on health literacy*. Ottawa, ON: Canadian Public Health Association. Retrieved from http://www.cpha.ca/uploads/portals/h-l/report_e.pdf

Schwarz, G., & Crenshaw, C. (2011). Old media, new media: The graphic novel as bildungsroman. *Journal of Media Literacy Education, 3*(1), 47–53.

Tran-Nguyen, B., Van Acken, L., Haberlin, Q., Coe, S., & Dunn-Krahn, S. (2013). *Chasing Adland.* Victoria, BC: D. Begoray, J. Wharf Higgins, & UVic Centre for Youth & Society. Available from http://www.gvpl.ca/ assets/PDF/Audiences/Teens/Chasing-Adland.pdf

Viner, R. M., Ozer, E. M., Denny, S., Marmot, M., Resnick, M., Fatusi, A., & Currie, C. (2012). Adolescence and the social determinants of health. *The Lancet, 379*(9826), 1641–1652.

Weber, K., Story, M., & Harnack, L. (2006). Internet food marketing strategies aimed at children and adolescents: A content analysis of food and beverage brand web sites. *Journal of the American Dietetic Association, 106*(9), 1463–1466.

Weintraub Austin, E., & Hust, S. (2005). Targeting adolescents? The content and frequency of alcoholic and nonalcoholic beverage ads in magazine and video formats November 1999–April 2000. *Journal of Health Communication: International Perspectives, 10*(8), 769–785.

Wharf Higgins, J., & Begoray, D. (2012). Exploring the borderlands between media and health: Conceptualizing 'Critical Media Health Literacy.' *Journal of Media Literacy Education, 4*(2), 136–148.

Wharf Higgins, J., Begoray, D., & MacDonald, M. (2009). A social ecological conceptual framework for understanding adolescent health literacy in the health education classroom. *American Journal of Community Psychology, 44*(3–4), 350–361.

World Health Organization. (2011). *Social determinants approaches to public health: From concept to practice*. Geneva, Switzerland: Author.

Yin, R. K. (2009). *Case study research: Design methods* (4th ed.). Thousand Oaks, CA: SAGE.

In: Adolescent Health Literacy and Learning
Editors: D. L. Begoray and E. M. Banister
ISBN: 978-1-63482-897-0

Chapter 4

HIGH SCHOOL HEALTH LITERACY IN BURMA/MYANMAR

***Christine Beer*[*,1] *and Deborah Begoray*[2]**
[1]Independent Researcher, IBM Global Business Services and Gevity, Canada
[2]Department of Curriculum and Instruction, University of Victoria, Canada

ABSTRACT

The purpose of this research was to examine health literacy in a high school in Yangon, Burma/Myanmar. Students were engaged in an interdisciplinary curriculum project with the purpose of exploring mental health issues. Data were collected in face-to-face and online social media learning environments and from web media that was accessed and/or created by the students. Data analysis used the concept of critical media health literacy, a theoretical model of health promotion that suggests the use of critical literacy to deal with media and consumer risk, leading to empowered citizenship. Students responded in varying ways to their exploration of mental health. Three major themes emerged: optimism, anxiety, and taking control. Two major conclusions were reached: such curricular activities can help students to engage in questions of mental health and contextual factors need to be added to a theoretical model of critical media health literacy.

Keywords: high school, Burma, Myanmar, mental health, social media

INTRODUCTION

Focusing Questions

1. What mental health issues do you think are of importance to high school age adolescents?

---

[*] Correspondence to (email): beercm@gmail.com

2. What do you see as the strengths and challenges of using technology in adolescent health literacy education?

The World Health Organization (WHO) defines health as "a state of complete physical, mental and social well-being and not merely the absence of disease or infirmity" (WHO, 2003). Adolescents around the world face several common challenges to their health: sedentary behaviours, stress, physical and psychological violence, and unsafe sexual reproductive health practices (WHO, 2014).

In Burma/Myanmar (n.b., we use Burma/Myanmar to recognize the contested usage of Burma versus Myanmar) where this study was conducted, rates of HIV/AIDS are higher in adolescent populations between the ages of 15 and 24 years than in populations between the ages of 25 and 49 (Asia Society, 2010). There is a risk that adolescent health challenges, when not effectively mitigated, will develop into chronic health problems.

Chronic health problems amongst adolescents everywhere have been shown to be related to interactions with online media. Adolescents around the globe are rapidly increasing their use of online media for communication and entertainment (Alpay, Verhoef, Xie, Te'eni, & Zwetsloot-Schonket, 2009; Marschollek, 2007). Online media consumption and interaction have direct and indirect influences on adolescent health literacy in terms of health beliefs, values, and health performances (Rootman, Frankish, & Kaszap, 2007; Wharf Higgins & Begoray, 2012). These trends suggest that school-based health literacy curricula need to reflect the importance of online, socially determined contexts in order to help adolescents improve their health (Young, Leger, & Blanchard, 2013).

Socially Determined Contexts

The notion of socially determined contexts (Martinko & Gardner, 1987) posits that the individual and collaborative psychological activities of human beings are mediated by contextualized signs and tools that are socially constructed (Birenbaum, 2003). For example, signs (e.g., images and written language) have contextualized meanings based on the social and cultural experiences of the audience; these signs are reproduced, recreated, and repeated as messages by using tools such as online social media. Social media is designed based on the beliefs and values of the designers who present and receive signs. For example, Facebook™ and Twitter™ are socially constructed and offer structures such as profiles and updates that can be manipulated by users and are in turn understood by others as worthy of comment or not. Users may choose to misrepresent themselves, and readers decide to believe or disbelieve such representations. Many social messages pertain to health directly or indirectly; for example, users may report on alcohol consumption, feelings of sadness and so on. Curricula on health literacy must be designed to guide adolescents to explore how (a) their own beliefs and intentions about health relate to and are influenced by the social constructions of media, and (b) they might become more active responders to these messages. Indeed, researchers have pointed to a need for health literacy concepts to explain empowerment and social participation (Wharf Higgins & Begoray, 2012; Zarcadoolas & Pleasant, 2009) as skills that can be learned by adolescents to inform and influence wellbeing in socially determined contexts.

Health literacy learning for adolescents requires curricula and educators that help adolescents to reflect upon and negotiate health knowledge in socially determined contexts. There is, however, a lack of data to explain why some adolescents are more successful negotiating their own wellbeing (Blakemore, 2012), understanding how their social contexts influence them, and in turn changing their socially determined contexts. Wellbeing can be threatened by mental health issues (e.g., vulnerability, depression, anxiety and eating disorders) which are present in socially determined contexts. These mental health issues increase steeply during adolescence (Paus, Keshavan, & Giedd, 2008). The issues may, in part, be brought on by adolescents comparing themselves unfavourably with others in various social contexts, both face to face and online. There is, therefore, a need for school-based health literacy curricula to help adolescents explore social contexts and threats to wellbeing. Such curricula are necessary to help adolescents improve their health outcomes, especially those associated with mental health.

In this study, participants described mental health issues as events that caused them *stress*. The health literacy curriculum used in this study was designed to guide an exploration of and skills acquisition for, first, consuming and creating web media content on stress and, second, interacting with emerging social media technologies to promote empowerment and control over stress.

Health Literacy as Sociocultural Basis for Research with Adolescents

No research on adolescent behaviours can proceed without taking into account the characteristics of this developmental stage. The unique assumptions, circumstances, and organization of socially determined contexts, including those mediated by online social media, affect the social and physiological transitions of adolescence. Health literacy is a personal capacity shaped by conditions in which a person lives and by the distribution of economic and political resources at local and global levels (WHO, 2013). Positioning health literacy as a social determinant of health suggests that adolescents have opportunities to construct health meanings and performances while participating in their various sociocultural contexts (Vygotsky, 1978), including their role as citizens now and as future adults (Wharf Higgins & Begoray, 2012).

Citizenship is a practice of evaluation and decision-making in situations where a person must reflect upon, critique, and negotiate conflicting views in order to achieve a healthy and just society (Wharf Higgins & Begoray, 2012). Social learning processes support students in their development of critical capacities and construction of meanings (Brown & Adler, 2008) as well as have potential for adolescents to learn and practice citizenship. The construction of meanings through social learning can allow students to learn how to critically inquire into the nature and operation of ideological, technological, and economic power and then, in turn, to work for change or elimination of oppressive situations (Freire, 2000; Giroux, 2005). Researchers have shown that social learning processes that engage adolescents to practice such citizenship help adolescents develop self-efficacy in their citizenship practices (Serek, Lacinová, & Macek, 2012). There appears to be a synergistic relationship between adolescents' critical evaluation and decision-making skills and their capacity for self-efficacy.

Adolescents' development of self-efficacy is enhanced by a learned capacity for self-determination that is characterized by autonomy, competence, and relatedness (Ryan & Deci, 2000). Competence is conceptualized as an experience of effectively bringing about desired outcomes and is associated with feelings of autonomy and wellbeing in relation to the self and teacher (Ryan, Patrick, Deci, & Williams, 2008). Relatedness, self-efficacy, and citizenship are necessary components of health literacy theory if health literacy theory is to be effectively applied in school-based curricula. These components support the ability of adolescents to (a) evaluate the consequences of their behaviours, (b) evaluate the relevance of health issues, and (c) achieve an intended positive health performance outcome (Paakkari & Paakkari, 2012). Self-efficacy and self-determination are, therefore, critical capacities of empowerment and attributes of citizenship. They also form the basis of the concept of critical media health literacy (CMHL,Wharf Higgins & Begoray, 2012).

CMHL is a three-concept process model that networks the attributes of skill, empowerment, and engaged citizenship for exploring how individuals "critically interpret and use media as a means to engage in decision-making processes and dialogues; exert control over their health and everyday events; and make healthy changes for themselves and their communities" (Wharf Higgins & Begoray, 2012, p. 142). The CMHL model calls for a transformative pedagogy in which educators work with adolescents as participants in research and in the design of curriculum to explore how health literacy is acquired through their experiences and how that experiential knowledge serves or does not serve their health performance outcomes. As the conceptual framework for the case study described below, CMHL was utilized for both the research and design of the interdisciplinary curriculum as a way to situate adolescents to explore mental health issues and to help positively influence their health outcomes.

It is particularly important to note that the location of this study was a high school in Yangon, Burma/Myanmar. This research environment helps to accentuate the importance of the context to any concept of health literacy for adolescents.

Observations of Yangon, Burma/Myanmar

Yangon is a city where contrasts abound. Many of the people who walk and ride their bicycles amongst the congested and discordant traffic talk on cell phones, which operate on government-censored telecommunication and Internet services. While the population has access to some contemporary tools, citizens of Burma/Myanmar are the poorest in Asia due in large part to an underdeveloped economy and government corruption. Over four million people live in the city of Yangon, a majority without adequate drinking water, shelter, or energy resources. Of the Burmese population, 30% are estimated to have incomes below the threshold necessary to provide for basic needs such as food, sanitation, and health care; in the frontiers of Burma/Myanmar, 50% of the population lack income necessary for basic needs (Asia Society, 2010). People with luxury cars often have smart phones, laptops, and a range of global telecommunication services because of business relationships with the military dictatorships that have controlled Burma since 1962 (British Broadcasting Company, 2015).

Burma was isolated from the international community by the ruling military juntas from 1962 to 2011; in 2011, the military began directing a transition to representative government. This process has not been without challenges and setbacks. Nevertheless, equity and social justice are principles of the current democratic movement. In April 2012, Aung San Suu Kyi, an opposition politician and chairperson of the National League for Democracy in Burma/Myanmar, was elected to a representational seat in the dictatorship's emerging parliamentary-style government. She is a powerful role-model who exemplifies the shared responsibilities and duties of citizenship to improve social and economic circumstances for people in Burma/Myanmar. Social and economic circumstances (e.g., health, housing, water and energy resources, income level, education level, social support) have major impacts on the health of people living in Yangon. Income levels are low for the majority of the estimated 60 million people who live in Burma/Myanmar; only foreigners and a small percentage of Burmese have access to wealth. Wealth in Yangon is defined as income that affords adequate food, shelter, safety, education, health care, and transportation. Higher income levels result generally in better physical health, access to K–12 education, and safer housing. The houses in which most participants of this case study lived are similar in appearance and scale to those in suburban areas of Canada or the United States but with their own oil-burning electricity generators and drinking water systems due to the lack of adequate public utility and water infrastructure. Participants' health services were provided by traditional Chinese practitioners and the few private clinics in Yangon, complemented by access to private Western-style medical practitioners in Bangkok and Singapore. During a year in Yangon, the first author observed that most of the participants travelled several times per year outside of Burma/Myanmar (e.g., other Southeast Asian countries and Europe) and were influenced by both their local Burmese and globalized Western concepts of health.

At the international high school where this case study was conducted, courses were taught in English; however, Burmese was spoken almost exclusively by Burmese staff and by the students when they were not in taking part in a class. Local cultural beliefs, values, and motivations were present in the school's social structures. For example, during a teacher orientation, a female Burmese teaching assistant leading the orientation explained to the foreign teachers that males have more value than females. She illustrated her point with this example: if her son was lying on the floor in her house playing video games and she needed to walk past him, she could not step over him but must instead walk around him so she would not be "above" him. Most students at the high school had smart phones and laptops to access the Internet for personal entertainment, communication, and school projects. Entertainment was described by the adolescent participants of this case study mainly in terms of the use of online social media including the use of Facebook, blogs, gaming, and videos.

It was common for participants to have multiple accounts in social media products. For example, one participant stated that she has two Facebook accounts with different photos and names. The photos and names were not her own. Her online personas, including photos she appropriated from the Web, were in sharp contrast to her actual appearance, age, interests, and in-class personality. She described her Facebook wall postings and emails as a form of fictional play in which she adopted the role of a globalized adult.

Facebook was also popular for accessing online video games, in which the Burmese students played roles in artificial battlefields and other social contexts. Many students had their own technology in their homes (e.g., Xbox™ consoles) for battlefield and race car games as well as digital video equipment and software for creating and editing movies. Amongst the array of digital and online entertainment, one of the most popular formats for male students was massively multiplayer online role-playing games (MMORPG), especially *World of Warcraft*©. Participants exploited an ever-growing array of online media to entertain themselves, communicate with each other, and create new content. This was an ideal environment to explore students' CMHL.

A Case Study of CMHL and Burmese High School Students

There is a lack of research on adolescent health in Burma/Myanmar despite the country having one of the highest disease burdens of tuberculosis, HIV infections, and AIDS-related deaths. This disease burden is due in part to limited development of health and education systems (Grundy, Annear, Ahmed, & Biggs, 2014). A report supported by the Myanmar Ministry of Health indicates that most adolescents in Burma/Myanmar misunderstand the risks and prevention of HIV (WHO, 2015). Looking to the broader geographical area of Southeast Asia, we know that adolescents also face significant health risks in the areas of violence and mental health (WHO, 2014).

Mental and physical health is an important foundation for the social participation in societal concerns. Researchers focused on Burmese youth and democratic citizenship (e.g., James, 2005) warn that the education system in Burma/Myanmar is not meeting the needs of youth to develop the critical capacities for active participation as citizens in a healthy public life. While aid organizations develop programs to reduce health risks in Burma/Myanmar, there appears to be a lack of health-promotion programming to engage adolescents in processes of citizenship to explore and overcome barriers to better health.

Considering the adolescents' health challenges combined with their intensive and increasing use of online social media and changing sociopolitical situation, there was cause for considerable concern about adolescent health literacy in Burma/Myanmar. The international high school where this case study was situated had a mission statement that considered critical thinking, the development of healthy lifestyles, and the role of technology in student learning across all subjects to be valued components of the curriculum, which seemed to support the purpose of the case study: researching the critical media health literacy of students. Due to the lack of health literacy research specific to Burmese adolescents, we looked to the broader international community for examples of health literacy research. Research in settings in Taiwan, Israel, The Netherlands, and Canada showed that health literacy interventions help adolescents affect their health status and outcomes (Levin-Zamir, Lemish, & Gofin, 2011; Li-Chun, 2010; Simovska, 2012; Wharf Higgins, Begoray, & MacDonald, 2009). Yet these studies also reported that the high school health education curriculum was often neither designed nor facilitated to engage adolescents with the critical processes and the socially determined media contexts relevant to adolescents' health. We, therefore, sought to develop a health literacy curriculum and to study students' responses to that curriculum.

Conceptual Orientation of the Case Study

The conceptual orientation of this case study drew upon the work of earlier researchers, in particular, on the three-concept process model of CMHL (Wharf Higgins & Begoray, 2012). The research question for this work was: How is CMHL expressed by high school students situated in Burma/Myanmar?

Research Procedures and High School Interdisciplinary Curriculum

We collected data through interviews (Appendix A) with participants and observations. Interviews provided information about the social backgrounds of participants, a sampling of participants' health concerns, and relevance of CMHL to the participants. Open-ended questions were based on the concepts of health literacy, media health literacy, and CMHL. Participants ($N = 20$) were recruited from an interdisciplinary health literacy and technology course of the international high school. The students were aged 15–18 years; 10 were girls and 10 were boys; 18 were Burmese and Chinese with the remaining two from Singapore and Thailand. The first author was the designer and instructor of the interdisciplinary course. Following a presentation and discussion of research data about adolescent health and health literacy during the first session, students brainstormed and voted on a health theme for the course. The topic *mental health* was chosen by the students for online blog discussions, web page designs, and face-to-face group discussions. For the web page designs, each student was encouraged to choose a particular area of interest related to the topic of mental health. Participants were provided with a web page design rubric (Appendix B) covering the technology and graphic design requirements as well as open-ended questions to guide exploration and development of health literacy. Each participant presented a web page design and helped to facilitate a discussion about the web page and online inquiry into their chosen mental health issue. The discussions were based on a focus group format (Yin, 2012) in which all students in the course had opportunities to ask questions, comment, and critique web page designs.

In support of participants' online inquiries, the online blog was guided by a protocol (Yin, 2012) consisting of seven questions: Do you think about your mental health? How do you think your ideas of mental health are affected by your friends and family? How do you think your ideas about mental health are affected by your online reading and conversations, such as on news websites or Facebook? How do you decide which information to use from websites? Have you ever decided to change your behaviour because of something you saw in a website, television program, movie, or sports event? If so, why did you try to change? All interviews and blogs were transcribed for analysis. Interview transcripts, samples of writing, and web pages were coded using an open coding process (Stake, 1995). After the first stage of encoding, each topically coded segment was grouped into one or more generalized categories, and then categorically organized segments were grouped into one or more themes, which are presented below.

FINDINGS

Three Themes: Optimism, Anxiety, and Taking Action

Analysis of the data revealed three major themes: optimism, anxiety, and taking action. *Optimism* is a confident attitude about mental health and future conditions of health, *anxiety* are feelings of uncertainty and unease about health, and *taking action* are plans to change in order to improve health.

Optimism

Optimism was observed as a state of confidence in mental health. In some instances, participants based their ideas about health on Burmese beliefs. One student described his concept of health as *a happy background and environment, peace* and said that his enjoyment of playing sports was based on his self-identified position as a Buddhist who sees health as *why we're here. God made us. It's essential.* Social media was frequently described as a source of happy feelings and relationships. One student posted to the blog that she *felt happy whenever good news* was posted to Facebook.

On a web page design, a student described his positive feelings about his role in online activities as a *first person shooter* in a MMORPG, an activity that connects players from around the world and, for him, takes *every second of attention and ... will result in a happy day.*

Happy results were described in a web page design demonstrating a student's attitude toward dealing with stress that she saw as unique to adolescents. Her messages conveyed her belief that the power to *help yourself* is a feature of mental health. Her design demonstrated her belief that she and others like her had power to influence future mental health conditions. She advised readers, *You can either change your situation or change your reaction ... focus on what makes you feel calm and in control.* Her comment conveys a hopefulness and confidence that she and her peers can positively influence their mental health and the contexts in which they are situated.

Anxiety

Anxiety was described by participants as a sense of unease and uncertainty about mental health outcomes, usually as a result of relationship difficulties. For example, a student described on the blog that he had relocated with his family many times and as a result felt *isolated and* [was] *having a breakdown.*

Anxiety was also connected to depression. One student designed a web page to describe how he was *feeling kinda depressed* at the increased pressure on grades in high school. He told his peers, *My parents are only happy when I have A's.* A student added that the stress was increasing because, based on an informal survey of her friends, *seven out of nine students have two tuitions a day and they're three hours each.* Tuitions are after-school classes, often conducted in the homes of the students, in which Burmese tutors review school subjects and prepare the students to take university entrance examinations. Several students said that they were *sharing this academic stress.*

Data showed a prevalence of uncertainty about the use of online media. In a blog describing anxiety about Facebook posts, one student commented, *As everyone knows, Facebook isn't a trustworthy webpage ... Facebook is like a page where people spread all the rumors, bad things, good things and nearly everything.*

The comment that Facebook is not trustworthy appears here to indicate it was not designed to be good or bad but as a structured social media tool separate from the good and bad messages that are conveyed through it. Another student posted on the blog, *Facebook ... affects your mental health both positively and negatively,* and then expressed anxiety as she noted, *Facebook users ... humiliated or made fun of by other people,* [who have] *fake profiles* [and cause] *harm.* Such comments convey a belief that Facebook as a technological tool is neutral and it is the way the tool is used that causes anxiety-promoting content.

Taking Action

Taking action was observed as ways of advocating for individual agency to improve one's mental health. When asked how social media influenced changes to health performances, a student described her motivation to avoid social interactions that were harmful to her emotional health. Another student explained that her motivation to take action through a change in health performance was based on her belief that any action is an improvement over inaction. She said, *Yes, I have. I tried to change because I wanted to know if it will work and I thought that it will be better than not doing anything*.

At times, the basis for behaviour change was not critically evaluated by participants. For example, Facebook was personified by one student as a super peer (Brown, Halpern, & L'Engle, 2005); that is, a knowledgeable and friendly influencer, worthy of trust: *Facebook works very efficiently in updating us on mental health issues, mainly because all topics and issues can be discussed quite openly. Be it a wall post, link, image, or even a chat*. Google™ was also described as a source for believable information. Indeed, search engines such as Google are designed to work in certain ways to privilege some sources over others (Hargittai, 2007). Most participants habitually utilized *the links at the top of the Google page* that were presented after a search, and then decided what to use based on what they called the *little descriptions* under the hyperlinks on the first page of the search results, ignoring search results beyond the first page. Google served as an influential super peer, leading them to information upon which to act.

For the participants, taking action was based on the believability of information and on repetition: *I chose to use the information that is realistic and is seen in most of the health website because, if an information appears again, for me, I believe that the information is true*. Countering this view, one student urged critical thought before taking action; she posted on the blog, *Do you understand this idea? Do you think it is reliable?* Interestingly, no one responded to her critical questions. Students described their beliefs and motivations, yet their descriptions did not demonstrate a particular motivation to critically evaluate a concept or situation before taking action.

How Themes Relate to the Literature of Adolescent Health Literacy and Learning

Participants described their beliefs and motivations and revealed some aspects of CMHL (Wharf Higgins & Begoray, 2012). In particular, they demonstrated ways of critiquing health using skills of asking questions and assessing the validity of online information. Similar to findings in previous studies with adolescents, these students utilized the instructional activity to engage in dialogue with peers (Larson, 2009) that appeared to help them critique the sociocultural conditions of health (Woodgate & Leach, 2010).

Anxiety described by the participants is similar to that reported in previous studies that adolescents' physiological and socially transitional experiences have a significant bearing on their perceptions of anxiety in social contexts (Paus et al., 2008; Rogoff, 2003; Steinberg, Vandell, & Bornstein, 2011). Ironically, it appears that participants were motivated by anxiety to change or control social relationships in order to manage physical or mental health and, thus, take action. Optimism appears as a passive acceptance of life events or a result of the ability to respond to social determinants of health and seek positive activities. Previous research indicates that adolescent autonomy is connected to a sense of competence for responding to social determinants of health (Woodgate & Leach, 2010) and achieving desired outcomes (Reis, Sheldon, Gable, Roscoe, & Ryan, 2000; Skinner, Furrer, Marchand, & Kindermann, 2008).

Information transmission, conversations, and activities conducted via social media were discussed by participants as a source of both optimism and anxiety. Similar to findings in previous research with adolescents, the processes of accepting transmitted content contrasted with how adolescents utilize critical literacy skills. Critical literacy skills for understanding content and implications of activities depends on the adolescents' capacity to negotiate for their own wellbeing (Li-Chun, 2010; Steinberg et al., 2011), to reflect on their perceptions of media as a super peer (Brown et al., 2005), and to engage in patterns of participation in relationships and learning situations involving socially determined contexts (Simovska, 2012).

Online social media was described by participants as an inevitable part of adolescent life, offering both a source of optimism and anxiety and a way to express their ideal selves. There was, however, little evidence to show that critical engagement was valued or enacted within socially determined contexts such as online gaming communities. Kress (2011) argued that representational modes and existing multimodal texts are unique to a "social group and its cultures at a particular moment [and constitute] distinct resources for making meaning" (p. 242). Critique as a way for making meaning appeared to be bypassed by participants due to either the power of a mode or multimodal text to which the viewer feels a strong need for identification (e.g., online gaming) or the lack of ability to critique online textual communications and content.

Some participants showed a worrisome willingness to accept, without a process of evaluation or questioning, health information that is presented by a source seen as authoritative (e.g., Google). In addition, they seemed to be willing to take action based on this frequently flawed, or at least unexamined, information. The increased likeliness of accessing online content related to health (Alpay et al., 2009; Li-Chun, 2010) was apparent for these participants. Similar to findings from previous research with high school students, content from media was also read in ways that influence health (Begoray, Cimon, & Wharf Higgins, 2010; Levin-Zamir et al., 2011). For example, characters on a television program who drink alcohol excessively without any negative consequences constitutes a dangerous health message for viewers. The media, it seems, is a health educator (Begoray et al., 2010; O'Keefe & Clarke-Pearson, 2011) and not one we might choose to be of such importance in the lives of adolescents.

LIMITATIONS OF THE STUDY

The unique needs of this Burmese population require further exploration. For example, this case study did not uncover knowledge about the participants' motivations and capacities for understanding and critiquing how the contexts of their socioeconomic and physical environments influence their health. Furthermore, the study did not uncover knowledge about motivation and capacities for taking action that engages with their broad range of socially determined contexts. The findings, nevertheless, suggest the need for a health literacy curriculum that facilitates an exploration of how opposing social authorities, or power, in socially determined contexts (e.g., Facebook or a Google source) relates to the changing roles and potential roles of these adolescents as citizens. They will become adults and the healthy future of Burma may depend in part on their ability to negotiate for their own wellbeing and the wellbeing of their communities. The themes of optimism, anxiety, and taking action are drawn from descriptions of the participants' interactions in social contexts involving a variety of roles and positions of power. In particular, there is a lack of data from this case study to explain how online media — whether as a political instrument of government or an online game — objectify the participants or allow individuals as citizens to take action and transform social contexts that are subtly, indirectly, or overtly oppressive (Giroux, 2005). Ultimately, all of these questions have a bearing on adolescent health.

IMPLICATIONS FOR RESEARCH AND PEDAGOGY

In this study, skills for understanding, interpreting, and reflecting on information appear to be based on personal reflection and motivation for helping peers with mental health. Explicit practice of skills for understanding, interpreting, and reflecting on information influenced some participants to take action based on their experiences of anxiety and optimism; in turn, their exploration of anxiety and optimism led to the development of more skills (e.g., those needed to create web sites and multimodal texts). The synergistic relationships between skills and inquiries into mental health were expressed from particular identities in socially determined contexts. This finding suggests that these students — like adolescents in other settings discussed in the literature (e.g., Levin-Zamir et al., 2011; Serek et al., 2012) — are enacting identities. Nevertheless, questions are left unanswered: What identities are enacted through social media? How are identities conceptualized and negotiated in relation to the nondigital self and socially determined contexts? Why are social media structures and messages perceived as immutable?

The themes of this study uncovered expressions of anxiety but also of optimism and empowerment in which the students could take action and make informed decisions to enhance their own health. Yet there is a lack of evidence to show how they might learn to interact through social media to advocate for structural changes to enhance personal health or the health of a social group (Dredze, 2012), which is vitally important for a country such as Burma/Myanmar. Some questions remain: What possibilities for empowerment do social, and social media, roles and identities provide for individuals to critically interact with socially determined contexts to improve health performance outcomes? How do identities empower individuals to engage their own personal characteristics (e.g., gender) to take health-promoting action in their social environments?

SUGGESTIONS FOR FUTURE RESEARCH

In order to explore these questions, future research designs to investigate CMHL in adolescence would require more in-depth and longitudinal interview and observation processes to collect both quantitative and qualitative data. Quantitative data are needed to describe in detail the social determinants of health present in Burma/Myanmar; qualitative data are required to understand the conceptual variations of health literacy and socially determined contexts, including online media that are mediating factors and should be represented in measurement instruments (McCormack, Rush, Kandula, & Paasche-Orlow, 2011). Both quantitative and qualitative data are required to describe how existing theories of self-determination — described by autonomy, competence, and relatedness (Ryan & Deci, 2000) — support research with adolescents who are situated in Burma/Myanmar. Pre and post structured interviews would provide benchmarks for reporting on applicability of existing concepts to all adolescents, the variations present in Burma/Myanmar and in online media contexts, and changes to health literacy capacities over a multiyear study.

Variations in the dimensions of citizenship need to be specified into roles that suit unique research contexts. The findings of this study indicate that the role of *citizen* varies with contexts; for example, the hesitance of students to participate in a vote on themes for the health literacy curriculum suggests the definition of citizenship was more influenced by obedience to authority than by participation in a democratic process. There were opportunities for the participants of this study to define roles of citizenship appropriate to their high social and economic status, to achieve their desired health performance outcomes, and to become aware of more vulnerable peers. Critique is a process that originates in a person's concept of the self in roles and contexts, where both roles and contexts hold affordances for power to taking action for the self or a community (Giroux, 2005).

Participants in this study demonstrated that they were interested in taking action and were capable of accessing, consuming, and understanding a significant amount of online, health-related media content. But their understanding of content appeared to be primarily driven by their belief that they should understand the content in a certain way as a member of an identifiable social group. Concepts of health literacy need to support dimensions of critique that can be the basis of questions about identity positions (Seaman & Rheingold, 2013) as they relate to the development of health literacy capacities. How are particular online social media texts designed to be understood, and how does that designed intent potentially impact the health concepts and outcomes of adolescents? What online media resources hold authority in motivating adolescents' enactment of health performances? How do the modes and multimodal components of online textual resources influence the skills that adolescents actively use to develop health literacy? How does health knowledge appear differently in different online media modes?

In order to take up future research, a theoretical model is needed that defines a language for explaining how socially determined contexts mediate the health literacy practices of individuals who participate in those contexts. One alternative is to consider dimensions such as the system of relationships among skills, empowerment, and citizenship. It may be through an understanding of how adolescents negotiate the system of relations among the politics, economies, and cultures of socially determined contexts and the enactment of skills, empowerment, and citizenship that research could uncover how health performances of particular adolescent populations are contingent to the system of relationships. If contingencies in taking action in health performances are discovered by adolescents to be mutable or ahistorical, then they may be empowered to take action for themselves and others in their sociocultural contexts. A conceptual framework for future research based on CMHL (Figure 1) depicts suggested dimensions for a conceptual framework of future research designs.

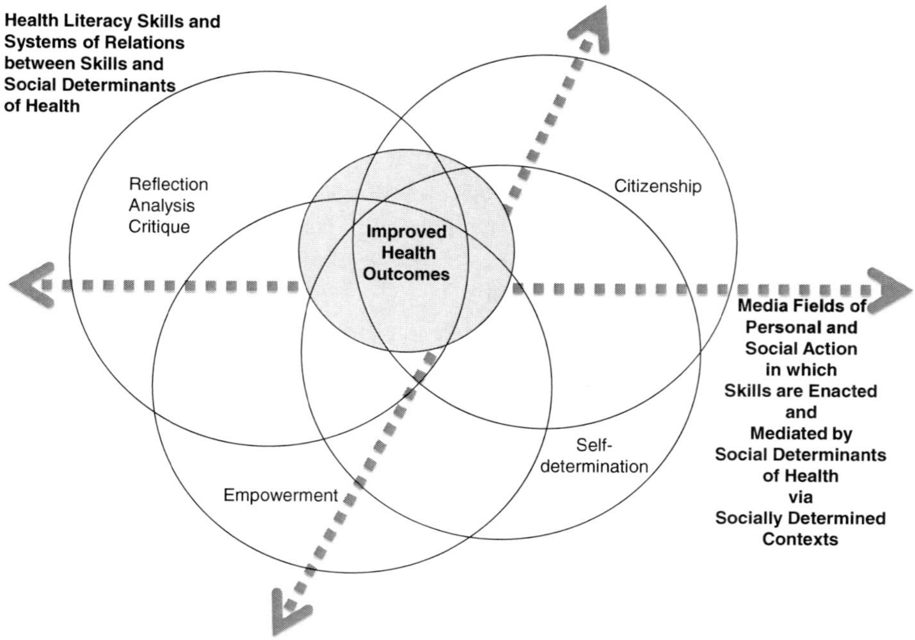

Figure 1. A conceptual framework for future research based on critical media health literacy (Wharf Higgins & Begoray, 2012).

The suggested conceptual framework shows the relationships between the development of skills for reflection, analysis, and critique and the development of capacities for empowerment, self-determination, and citizenship. Such skills and capacities are social determinants of health literacy and will lead to improved health performance outcomes. The social determinants of health literacy are framed by adolescents' participation in media fields, and the media fields are framed within socially determined contexts. Thus, the CMHL model of Wharf Higgins and Begoray (2012) is extended by this model. The suggested framework presents a multidimensional network of social determinants of health literacy and the social determinants of health mediated by socially determined contexts. The themes of this study show that anxiety, optimism, and taking action relate to these adolescents' skills for reflection, analysis, and critique and the development of capacities for empowerment, self-determination, and citizenship. The themes also indicate that socially determined contexts of online media are powerful influencers of health beliefs, values, and intentions to take action. In order to improve adolescent health literacy learning, adolescent health literacy research must examine how networks of the social determinants of health literacy, which can be learned, are mediated by the cross-section of social determinants of health and socially determined contexts.

CONCLUSION

Findings from this case study bring attention to the health literacy capacities and mental health needs of a group of high school students situated in Burma/Myanmar; it has offered an important window into an understudied population. Furthermore, the findings underline and suggest new lines of inquiry. Based on themes of the study, the Burmese adolescents' health literacy is influenced by a hybrid of their local Burmese-specific contexts and their online and in-school globalized contexts. Patterns of sensitivity to friends and peers, responses to online contacts, a need to feel in control of health, and a need to explore socially determined contexts related to health is a set of phenomena that corresponds to adolescents worldwide who are globalized by their online experiences. We note as well that the relative wealth of these adolescents did not protect them from mental health issues, which they seemed to share with adolescents in developed countries (e.g., Levin-Zamir et al., 2011).

Our findings indicate that CMHL translates to the particular context of this study and helps to explain adolescent health literacy capacities formed in relation to local Burmese contexts and globalized online contexts. When operationalized as curriculum, CMHL is shown as supportive of health literacy development of the adolescent participants in this study. Yet health literacy theory needs to continue to evolve in ways that explain and explore the relationships between adolescents' socially determined contexts and their beliefs and values that affect motivations and health performances.

It is significant that the findings from this case study showed few examples of critical engagement with power in socially determined contexts; however, the findings illustrate that many of these adolescents were highly motivated to overcome anxiety, be optimistic, and take control of their health. In addition, they demonstrated the capacity to ask questions and engage in dialogue to explore causal relationships that affect health, especially mental health. Clearly, there is an opportunity for further research to expand health literacy and engage adolescents in Burma/Myanmar and elsewhere with a school-based curriculum that helps them to improve their health outcomes.

Questions for Discussion, Reflection, and Writing

1. What did you find most surprising about the health concerns of these high school students?
2. Imagining you were a teacher or health worker dealing with this adolescent population, how might you seek to further develop their health literacy?
3. How do you see context as important to a theory of adolescent health literacy?

List of Online Resources

- New York City Department of Education: Student Social Media Guidelines – http://schools.nyc.gov/NR/rdonlyres/9765B2DF-9BD5-42AA-8D85-005D0FC8AA23/0/Student_Social_MediaGuidelines_finalv3_20140128.pdf
- Positive Mental Health Teacher Resources – http://www.everactive.org/positive-mental-health-teacher-resources

Appendix A. Open-Ended Questions Based on Theorists' Constructs of Health Literacy

Theorists	Constructs of health literacy	Research questions	Interview questions
Conceptual framework for critical media health literacy (Begoray et al., 2010, p. 26) Media health literacy (Levin-Zamir et al., 2011, p. 324)	Internal influences, personal and sociodemographic characteristics	1. What are the participants' demographic attributes?	a. What is your age? b. How long have you been attending this school? c. What is your nationality? d. What is your parents' ethnicity? e. What is your parents' education/profession? f. What is your living situation (e.g., with mother, with grandparents, independent)?
Conceptual model of health literacy as an asset (Nutbeam, 2008, p, 2076) Conceptual framework for critical media health literacy (Begoray et al., p. 26)	Developed knowledge and capability, participation in social norms and practices, changed health behaviours, attitudes, external influences, skills in identifying, understanding and assessing potential influence of health messages, self-reported health status, interacting with literacies situated in social contexts	2. What is the participants' knowledge of health?	a. How do you describe 'health'? Why? b. How do you describe your health? (At this point, begin replacing 'health' with descriptors given by interviewee if appropriate.) c. Do you think about your health? d. Do you think your ideas about health are affected by friends/family/media (e.g., information on the Internet or discussions on social websites)? If so, how? Why?
Media health literacy (Levin-Zamir et al., 2011, p. 324) New literacies (Lankshear & Knobel, 2011, p. 33)	Skills in negotiation and self-management, access, identify, understand, and assess influence of sources of health information, critique relevance to adolescence, interacting with literacies situated in social contexts	3. How do participants access, evaluate, and understand information about health?	a. How do you learn about health? b. Where does the information come from? c. How do you decide if the information is valid or important for you? d. How do you decide if the information is relevant for someone in your stage of life?
	Skills in social organization and advocacy for individual and community benefit, developed knowledge and capability to apply it, attitudes, communicate health messages, awareness of influence and intention to take action, interacting with literacies situated in social contexts	4. How do participants communicate about health and advocate for the benefit of their own health and the health of their friends and family?	a. If you learn something about a health issue, do you share it? If so, why? If so, how do you share it? b. Do you do anything differently because of what you learn? Why? c. How do you think you can influence your health? Why? d. Do you use what you learn to do anything on purpose to take care of your health? If so, how? Why? e. Do you think you have any influence over the health of friends/family members? If so, how? Why? f. Do you use what you learn to try to inform or influence friends/family members to do something about their health? If so, how? Why?

Appendix A. (Continued)

Theorists	Constructs of health literacy	Research questions	Interview questions
	Developed knowledge and capability to apply it, changed health behaviours, engagement in social action for health, participation in social norms and practices, attitudes, communicate, health empowerment, interacting with literacies situated in social contexts	5. What health outcomes have been realized by the participants as a result of their learning about health issues?	a. Have you learned anything in the past that helped you to do something about a personal health concern or issue? If so, what was it? b. Have you learned anything in the past that helped you to help a friend/family member with a health concern or issue? If so, what was it?
	Skills in negotiation and self-management, participation in social norms and practices, attitudes, identification, critical analysis, and awareness of the influences of health messages, interacting with literacies situated in social contexts	6. What external influences do the participants believe to be significant to their ideas and behaviours around health?	a. Who or what do you think influences your ideas of health? Why? b. What do you think makes you change your ideas of health? Why? c. What makes you change the things you do that affect your health? Why?

Appendix B. Webpage Design Rubric: A Webpage about a Health Issue

	Points (24 total possible)		
	1	2	3
Design	The webpage design is not entirely appropriate to the intended purpose and audience. The specific health topic is not expressed.	The webpage design is visually pleasing although it may not be entirely appropriate to the intended purpose or its intended audience. The health topic is clearly expressed with text or images.	The webpage design is visually pleasing, helps to deliver a specific health topic and purpose of the web page, and is appropriate for its intended audience. The site includes a way for readers to communicate online about the topic with the author or other readers.
Layout	The webpage layout is usable, but it has problems with clarity or placement of elements.	The webpage layout is largely effective although there may be some occasional problems with clarity or placement of elements.	The webpage uses an effective and uncluttered layout, using background to enhance the readability of text and the appearance of images, and users do not have to scroll to read the main contents.
Images	Several images on the webpage have problems with either design or mechanical presentation, and no images are original.	The images are well designed although there may be some minor problems with either design or mechanical presentation.	Most of the images are original and all images are well designed and mechanically effective, without distortion, excessive dithering, haloes, or other negative graphic effects.
Text	Text on the webpage has a problem with either style or mechanics or both, and no text or images are original.	Text on the webpage is readable and reasonably well written although there may be minor mechanical errors. The author has included text and images created by the author or remade from existing text and images.	Text on the page is well written and presented effectively, using readable fonts and text design and without major mechanical errors (e.g., grammar, punctuation, spelling), and most of the written text and images is the work of the webpage author.
Navigation	A reader can get around the webpage but only with some difficulty.	The webpage is well organized and easy to navigate for the most part with clear relationships between pages. Some sections may be more difficult to find or there may be links that do not lead anywhere.	The webpage is well organized and easy to navigate, links are appropriate, clearly labeled, and have a definite purpose.
Mechanics	The webpage includes either missing images or broken links. The webpage is not readable by Firefox or Explorer browsers.	The webpage includes either missing images or broken links. The webpage is readable by either Firefox or Explorer browsers.	Everything on the webpage works. There are no missing images or broken links, and the webpage can be read with Firefox or Explorer browsers.
HTML, XHTML, CSS	The XHTML/HTML code has incorrect or unnecessary tags, lacks proper nesting of tags, and repeated tags. The webpage does not use CSS elements to control design, content, and layout.	The XHTML/HTML code is largely clean although there may be a few questionable tags. The webpage uses CSS elements to control some portions of design, content, and layout.	The XHTML/HTML code is clean, without misused tags. Tags are nested and complete, a minimum of tags are used (use one tag with several attributes instead of repeated tags), header tags are used as headers. The webpage name, including folders, pages, images, and frames use lowercase text with no spaces. The webpage consistently uses CSS elements to control design, content, and layout.
Credibility	Webpage leaves user wondering about the origin and sources of its text and images.	Webpage includes author, date created or updated, and no copyright infringement.	Author names, affiliations, and credentials are included for all content; and the text explicitly states point of view. It is easy to identify original content, and material that is not the work of the webpage author includes appropriate citations with no copyright infringement. Site includes date created or updated.

REFERENCES

Alpay, L., Verhoef, J., Xie, B., Te'eni, D., & Zwetsloot-Schonk, J. H. M. (2009). Current challenges in consumer health informatics: Bridging the gap between access to information and information understanding. *Biomedical Informatics Insights, 2*, 1–10.

Asia Society. (2010). *Current realities and future possibilities in Burma/Myanmar: Options for U.S. policy.* New York, NY: Author. Retrieved from http://asiasociety.org /files/pdf/ASBurmaMyanmar_TaskForceReport.pdf

Begoray, D., Cimon, M., & Wharf Higgins, J. (2010). *Mediating health: The powerful role of media*. Hauppauge, NY: Nova Science.

Birenbaum, M. (2003). New insights into learning and teaching and their implications for assessment. In M. Segers, F. Dochy, & E. Cascallar (Eds.), *Optimizing new modes of assessment: In search of qualities and standards* (pp. 13–36). Dordrecht, The Netherlands: Kluwer.

Blakemore, S-J. (2012). Development of the social brain in adolescence. *Journal of the Royal Society of Medicine, 105*, 111–116.

British Broadcasting Company. (2015). *Myanmar profile*. Retrieved from http://www.bbc.co.uk/news/world-asia-pacific-12990563

Brown, J. D., Halpern, C. T., & L'Engle, K. L. (2005). Mass media as a sexual super peer for early maturing girls. *Journal of Adolescent Health, 36*(5), 420–427.

Brown, J. S., & Adler, R. P. (2008). Minds on fire: Open education, the long tail, and learning 2.0. *EDUCAUSE Review, 43*(1), 16–32.

Dredze, M. (2012). How social media will change public health. *IEEE Intelligent Systems, 27*(4), 81–84. Retrieved from http://www.computer.org/csdl/mags/ex/2012/ 04/mex2012040081-abs.html

Freire, P. (2000). *Pedagogy of the oppressed* (30th anniversary ed., M. B. Ramos, Trans.). New York, NY: Continuum.

Giroux, H. A. (2005). *Schooling and the struggle for public life: Democracy's promise and education's challenge.* Herndon, VA: Paradigm.

Grundy, J., Annear, P., Ahmed, S., & Biggs, B-A. (2014). Adapting to social and political transitions: The influence of history on health policy formation in the Republic of the Union of Myanmar (Burma). *Social Science & Medicine, 107*, 179–188.

Hargittai, E. (2007). The social, political, economic, and cultural dimensions of search engines: An introduction. *Journal of Computer-Mediated Communication, 12*(3), 769–777.

James, H. (2005) *Governance and civil society: Education, health and environment in Myanmar.* London, England: RoutledgeCurzon.

Kress, G. (2011). Partnerships in research: Multimodality and ethnography. *Qualitative Research, 11*(3), 239–260.

Lankshear, C., & Knobel, M. (2011). *New literacies: Everyday practices and classroom learning*. Berkshire, England: Open University Press.

Larson, L. (2009). Reader response meets new literacies: Empowering readers in online learning communities. *The Reading Teacher, 62*(8), 638–648.

Levin-Zamir, D., Lemish, D., & Gofin, R. (2011). Media health literacy (MHL): Development and measurement of the concept among adolescents. *Health Education Research, 26*(2), 323–335.

Li-Chun, C. (2010). Health literacy, self-reported status and health promoting behaviours for adolescents in Taiwan. *Journal of Clinical Nursing, 20*, 190–196.

Marschollek, M. (2007). Advances in education and consumer health informatics: Findings from the section on education and consumer informatics. In A. Geissbuhler, R. Haux, & C. Kulikowski (Eds.), *IMIA Yearbook of Medical Informatics* (pp. 95–97). Retrieved from http://www.schattauer.de/de/magazine/uebersicht/zeitschriften-a-z/imia-yearbook/imia-yearbook-2007/issue/special/manuscript/8422/show.html

Martinko, M., & Gardner, W. (1987). The leader/member attribution process. *Academy of Management Review, 12*(2), 235–249.

McCormack, L., Rush, S., Kandula, N., & Paasche-Orlow, M. (2011). Health literacy research: Looking forward. *Journal of Health Communication, 16*(Suppl. 3), 5–8.

Nutbeam, D. (2008). The evolving concept of health literacy. *Social Science & Medicine 67*(1), 2072–2078.

O'Keefe, G. S., & Clarke-Pearson, K. (2011). Health: The impact of social media on children, adolescents, and families. *Pediatrics, 127*(4), 800–804.

Paakkari, L., & Paakkari, O. (2012). Health literacy as a learning outcome in schools. *Health Education, 112*(2), 133–152.

Paus, T., Keshavan, M., & Giedd, J. N. (2008). Why do many psychiatric disorders emerge during adolescence? *Nature Reviews Neuroscience, 9*(12), 947–957.

Reis, H. T., Sheldon, K. M., Gable, S. L., Roscoe, J., & Ryan, R. M. (2000). Daily well-being: The role of autonomy, competence, and relatedness. *Personality and Social Psychology Bulletin, 26*, 419–435.

Rogoff, B. (2003). *The cultural nature of human development*. New York, NY: Oxford University Press.

Rootman, I., Frankish, J., & Kaszap, M. (2007). Health literacy: A new frontier. In M. O'Neill, S. Dupéré, A. Pederson, & I. Rootman (Eds.), *Health promotion in Canada: Critical perspectives* (2nd ed., pp. 61–74). Toronto, ON: Canadian Scholars' Press.

Ryan, R. M., & Deci, E. L. (2000). Self-determination theory and the facilitation of intrinsic motivation, social development, and well-being. *American Psychologist, 55*, 68–78.

Ryan, R. M., Patrick, H., Deci, E. L., & Williams, G. C. (2008). Facilitating health behaviour change and its maintenance: Interventions based on self-determination theory. *European Health Psychologist, 10*(1), 2–5.

Seaman, J., & Rheingold, A. (2013). Circle talks as situated experiential learning: Context, identity, and knowledgeability in "learning from reflection." *Journal of Experiential Education, 36*(2), 155–174.

Serek, J., Lacinová, L., & Macek, P. (2012). Does family experience influence political beliefs? Relation between interparental conflict perceptions and political efficacy in late adolescence. *Journal of Adolescence, 35*, 577–586.

Simovska, V. (2012). Case study of a participatory health promotion intervention in school. *Democracy and Education, 20*(1), 1–10.

Skinner, E. A., Furrer, C., Marchand, G., & Kindermann, T. (2008). Engagement and disaffection in the classroom: Part of a larger motivational dynamic? *Journal of Educational Psychology, 100*(4), 765–781.

Stake, R. E. (1995). *The art of case study research.* Thousand Oaks, CA: SAGE.

Steinberg, L., Vandell, D. L., & Bornstein, M. H. (2011). *Development: Infancy through adolescence.* Belmont, CA: Wadsworth Cengage Learning.

Vygotsky, L. S. (1978). *Mind in society: The development of higher psychological processes.* Cambridge, MA: Harvard University Press.

Wharf Higgins, J., & Begoray, D. (2012). Exploring the borderlands between media and health: Conceptualizing 'Critical Media Health Literacy.' *Journal of Media Literacy Education, 4*(2), 136–148.

Wharf Higgins, J., Begoray, D., & MacDonald, M. (2009). A social ecological conceptual framework for understanding adolescent health literacy in the health education classroom. *American Journal of Community Psychology, 44*(3–4), 350–362.

Woodgate, R. L., & Leach, J. (2010). Youth's perspectives on the determinants of health. *Qualitative Health Research, 20*(9), 1173–1182.

World Health Organization. (2003). *WHO definition of health.* Geneva, Switzerland: Author. Retrieved from www.who.int/about/definition/en/print.html

World Health Organization. (2013). *Health literacy: The solid facts.* Geneva, Switzerland: Author. Retrieved from http://www.euro.who.int/__data/assets/pdf_file/0008/190655/e96854.pdf

World Health Organization. (2014). *Adolescents: Health risks and solutions* (Fact Sheet No. 345). Geneva, Switzerland: Author. Retrieved from http://www.who.int/mediacentre/factsheets/fs345/en/

World Health Organization. (2015). *The impact of chronic disease in Myanmar.* Geneva, Switzerland: Author. Retrieved from http://www.who.int/chp/chronic_disease_report/media/impact/myanmar.pdf

Yin, R. K. (2012). *Applications of case study research* (3rd ed.).Thousand Oaks, CA: SAGE.

Young, I., Leger, L., & Blanchard, C. (2013). Health-promoting schools: Working in partnership to address global needs, a collaboration leading to the production of practical tools for practitioners. *Global Health Promotion, 20*(Suppl. 4), 122–127.

Zarcadoolas, C., & Pleasant, A. (2009). Health literacy in the digital world. In J. Parker & E. Thorson (Eds.), *Health communication in the new media landscape* (pp. 303–321). New York, NY: Springer.

In: Adolescent Health Literacy and Learning
Editors: D. L. Begoray and E. M. Banister

ISBN: 978-1-63482-897-0

Chapter 5

TEACHING MIDDLE SCHOOL ADOLESCENTS TO CRITICALLY REFLECT ON THE INTERACTION OF GENDER WITH HEALTH ADVERTISING

Elizabeth Banister[1]* and Deborah Begoray[2]
[1]School of Nursing, University of Victoria, Canada
[2]Department of Curriculum and Instruction, University of Victoria, Canada

ABSTRACT

This chapter describes how a case study with adolescents (ages 12–14 years) created contexts of interaction and intersubjective knowledge to reveal and engage their critical thinking about gendered health messages in media advertising. We focus specifically on how our choice of data collection strategies offered a window to observe how gender and sex were enacted and contextualized by culture and social location of a middle school classroom. Students were taught how to use iMovie and Green Screen technology on iPads for creating 2-minute advertisements to market healthy extracurricular participation among peers. Students were supplied with art materials for creating stick puppets to represent themselves in their ads. Data were collected through individual and focus group interviews, participant observation, and examination of the stick puppets. Participants had an active role in creating knowledge about the topic of inquiry, in this case, an advertisement for a healthy activity. We observed the ways in which the adolescents performed gender and how their social context offered a segue into understanding how norms of adolescent masculinity and femininity reaffirm the heteronormativity of the school culture. We maintain that developing a greater understanding of the influence of gender on adolescent health will afford the development of gender-appropriate interventions that can serve to help improve health education, improve adolescent health literacy, and empower researchers to investigate adolescent health literacy more effectively.

Keywords: gendered health messages, critical reflection, media advertising

* Correspondence to (email): ebaniste@uvic.ca

Introduction

Focusing Questions

1. How can dialogue between middle school adolescents and teachers encourage critical reflection on the topic of gender in health advertising?
2. How can research activities help to develop adolescent critical media health literacy?

Adolescence is marked by physical and emotional transitions as young people seek autonomy and prepare for adulthood. Societal expectations for gender and age-related behaviours become increasingly distinguished by differing societal expectations for boys and girls (MacLean, Sweeting, & Hunt, 2010). During this time, they are subjected to health information from multiple sources including messages of the commercial media (Begoray, Wharf Higgins, Harrison, & Collins-Emery, 2013) — much of which is inaccurate and unhealthy (Scull, Malik, & Kupersmidt, 2014). Such information has health implications for adolescents by conveying negative, stereotypical messages, especially in the portrayal of unrealistic and unhealthy role models for both girls and boys (Begoray, Banister, Wharf Higgins, & Wilmot, 2015). Most consumer goods that target youth are marketed in highly gendered and often sexualised ways, reinforcing gender distinctions and pressuring youth to purchase goods or clothing in order to fit in with their peers (Morrow, 2006).

Recent research has demonstrated the effectiveness of media literacy interventions in mitigating the harmful influence of media on risky behaviours (Bergsma, 2011; Jeong, Cho, & Hwang, 2012). Specifically, critical media instruction promotes methods for reflection and inquiry (Rogow, 2011) including processes to question “what stories get told and to whose benefit” (Ashcraft, 2012, p. 600) in advertising. The creation and evaluation of their own compositions, such as public service announcements for peers, can provide a context for such reflection. These activities can also support adolescents’ development to more abstract thinking (Banister, Begoray, & Daly, 2011) and thus improve the analysis of gender in commercial advertising messages.

In this chapter, we describe how our case study with adolescents created “contexts of interaction and intersubjective knowledge” (Flecha, Pulido, & Christou, 2011, p. 253) to reveal and engage adolescents’ critical thinking about gendered health messages in media advertising. The study has been reported in detail elsewhere (Begoray et al., 2015). In this chapter, we focus more specifically on how our choice of data collection strategies offered a window to observe how gender and sex were enacted and “contextualized by culture and social location” (Bottorff, Oliffe, Kelly, & Chambers, 2011, p. 176) of a middle school classroom. We illustrate this through our use of specific examples from our research. To provide the context, we first discuss media literacy education, then the social construction of gender and identity, and finally the promotion of critical thinking.

Media Literacy and Health Education

A basic principle of media literacy education is that “teaching critical thinking skills creates an active filter through which media messages may be processed” (Scull et al., 2014,

p. 3) whereby students learn to "evaluate and critique the reality of media messages they create" (Rogow, 2011, p. 18). Importantly, they engage in dialogue and are open to shifts in perspective as they listen to each other's points of view (Rogow, 2011). Educators need to provide adolescents with multiple opportunities that inspire adolescents to "begin asking why?" (Oliver, 2001, p. 162).

We approached our study to be congruent with basic concepts of British Columbia's (BC) newly drafted English Language Arts Curriculum, Grade 8 (BC Ministry of Education [MOE], 2013a), which emphasizes "core competencies of thinking, communication and social and personal competencies [to] support lifelong learning" (n.p.). For example, that curriculum includes learning standards that students be able to "analyze the ways language can be manipulated for specific purposes including ways to evoke emotional responses, [examine] the accuracy, reliability, and relevance of information, [and] create a variety of texts to communicate ideas, create impact, and evoke emotion" (n.p.). In addition, the Grade 8 Physical and Health Education curriculum (MOE, 2013b) stipulates that students will comprehend "factors that influence personal health decisions, including the media and peers, … influences on individual identities, including sexual identity, gender, values, and beliefs, [and] safe use of the internet and social media" (n.p.). While we remained aware of curricular demands, we also wanted to add goals that brought together media literacy and health education, specifically addressing students' ability to critically question gender and identity messages of advertising.

Social Construction of Gender and Identity in Adolescents

We understand gender as "socially constructed, dynamic, and influenced by contextual factors, embedded in a multifaceted array of social factors underlying human experience" (Bottorff, Oliffe, & Kelly, 2012, p. 436). Individuals' learning about gender influences reflects their differing identity and self-presentation concerns (Manago, Graham, Greenfield, & Salimkhan, 2008). Adolescents use a range of evidence regarding gender roles including evidence from parents, individuals they observe around them, and through their understandings of the media (Francis as cited in Morrow, 2006). One study, for example, found that boys "typically report that they always have to be tough; watch themselves lest they appear too smart; and be careful not to do anything that could construed as 'gay' or 'girly'" (Caldwell, 2012, p. 9). Similarly, Thorne (as cited in Morrow, 2006) observed that boys tend to be subject to more rigid boundaries concerning gender behaviour and to policing by peers and adults should they show feminine qualities. Caldwell (2012) also found that girls struggle with "their feelings of being judged on looks alone; not 'fitting in' with media stereotypes; and a sense that they can never be thin enough, pretty enough or happy enough" (p. 9).

Gender identity and behaviours are created through social interaction and through individuals' perceived gender expectations, negotiation of identity (Manago et al., 2008), and perceptions of themselves as gendered beings and how they are judged as such by others (Johnson & Repta, 2012). "Gender identities develop within gendered societies, where the pressure to adopt the 'correct' and 'corresponding' gender according to presenting sex is strong" (Johnson & Repta, 2012, p. 24). This belief in turn shapes adolescent behaviour based on what they believe is acceptable for their particular gender (Johnson & Repta, 2012). Morrow (2006) noted that young people convey "fixed stereotypical views of gender differences" (p. 99) and actively construct and comprehend polar opposite categories of masculine and feminine.

Gender identity development is a central task for adolescents; however, broader contextual influences on gender identity such as media effects and popular culture are surprisingly understudied (Morrow, 2006; ter Bogt, Engels, Bogers, & Kloosterman, 2010). Some research points out research difficulties in investigations that seek also to shape young adolescents' engagement with consumer culture. Oliver's (2001) critical inquiry with Grade 8 girls examining portrayals of the female body in teen magazines describes some of the challenges participants demonstrated in trying to view themselves and other females outside stereotypical portrayals. For example, one girl was able to identify why she liked a picture of a girl wearing a bathing suit (the girl was thinner than she was) but was not able to identify the kinds of messages about girls' bodies that such images convey. Oliver concluded that the girls made only miniscule steps in critiquing stereotypical views of their bodies, possibly because they were being asked to defy "traditional cultural values and norms" (p. 155). Oliver further admitted the difficulty for educators with accessing the kind of language that would serve to allow them to align with girls in order to help the girls critique and examine an issue. She also contended that instructors need patience as girls "develop their critical capacities" (p. 162).

Others have noted the challenges with engaging adolescent participants with researchers' questions, particularly when asked to assume the subjectivity of "a perceived other" in terms of gender (Haines, Johnson, Carter, & Arora, 2009, p. 2035). These challenges are not surprising given that school contexts often serve to reinforce gender norms and behaviours and have direct consequences for those who transgress such norms (Haines et al., 2009; Morrow, 2006). In-school research interviews may suffer the same constraints. Interviews can serve as a performance of gender (Haines et al., 2009; Morrow, 2006); they are influenced by the social positioning of researchers and participants and how these interact to influence what and how much participants are willing to disclose (Archer, 2002). Haines et al. (2009) noted that "while age and gender dynamics may be inevitable when conducting research with adolescents, [researchers need to develop] creative and participant-driven methodologies that enable young people to reflect on and discuss gender as they define and experience it" (p. 2035).

Promoting Critical Thinking by Adolescents

We undertook a number of measures to increase the likelihood of reflection by adolescents. One of these approaches was to promote critical thinking. In a widely cited study, Facione (1990) said that critical thinking is needed for inquiry and thus vital not only for education but in adult life. Lipman (as cited in Weaver & Alvermann, 2000) defined critical thinking as "thinking that facilitates judgment because it relies on criteria, is self-correcting and is sensitive to context" (p. 116); this definition is particularly suitable for adolescents facing a rapidly changing social environment.

Young adolescents are becoming more able to reason abstractly but need a foundation on which to base their reflection such as a personal experience so that "learning becomes relevant" (Caldwell, 2012, p. 6). In the classroom, students can be offered group experiences on which to reflect, as we did in this research study. To encourage critical thinking, interviewers need to employ questioning and discussion strategies that will allow adolescents time to think. For adolescents, this task often means trying out ideas and observing the response of teacher and peers. The research setting needs to be a safe environment so as to encourage the sharing of nascent ideas and moving beyond these initial ideas to more critical thinking.

Promoting critical thinking in discussion with adolescents needs to feature questions for which the instructor does not have an answer. Our focus group research questions were, of course, just such questions. We were inquiring about students' use of advertising to focus on audiences of girls or boys and asking for their reactions and opinions.

In such a "discussion as inquiry … students become intellectual explorers with questions whose answers they do not know, and that might take them to terrain they had not realized existed" (Wolsey & Lapp, 2009, p. 373). These students formulated their answers in conversation with the interviewer and with their peers. Our study was developed to foster critical thinking during both learning and reflecting phases.

Overview of Study

Our case study (Yin, 2009) took place weekly over a 7-week period in a middle school classroom located in a mid-sized city on the west coast of Canada. Our intent was to explore how adolescents (ages 12–14 years) critically analyze and evaluate messages about gender and health in the commercial media and then create gendered health messages through a video production project as an innovative health promotion tool. Our female team of four interdisciplinary researchers had a smooth entry to the site due to our previous research at the school in which rapport and credibility as researchers had been established (Begoray, Wharf Higgins, & MacDonald, 2009). Six (two male and four female) graduate student research assistants were assigned to gender-matched groups to assist students with the technological aspects of creating their video advertisements and to record their observations.

Students were taught how to use *iMovie*™ and *Green Screen*™ technology on iPads for creating 2-minute advertisements to market healthy extracurricular participation among peers. Students were supplied with art materials for creating stick puppets to represent themselves in their ads. Data were collected through individual and focus group interviews, participant observation, and examination of the stick puppets.

Interviews As a Context to Encourage Critical Media Health Literacy

Individual Interviews

Following completion of their health advertisements, we conducted individual interviews with all participants. We used an interview guide to foster consistency across the interviews that included critical questions (Appendix A) related to the study. Using their puppet as a prompt, we began the interview by asking them to look at their puppet to talk about their own representation and to explain why they chose to show themself as they did. We then showed each participant the entire group of stick puppets after having placed them into two separate gender-specific groups (boys and girls). The puppets enabled a more concrete bridge for adolescents to use in order to discuss abstract concepts such as gender (Chabot & Shoveller, 2012); they also served to prompt and quickly focus discussion and allowed students to more readily compare representations across gender groups (MacLean et al., 2010). For example, we asked participants to describe the physical features of their puppet to access their views of how the media and gender stereotypes might have influenced their creations.

In the following extract from an interview, a boy (age 12) describes how he decided on a puppet used in his group's advertisement about joining the rugby team:

> Interviewer: What I wanted to ask you today, was, given that your group was making an advertisement to sell rugby to the rest of your schoolmates and to guys, in particular, when you were making these puppets, what were you thinking of for the facial features, for body weight, for height, use of colour hair? What went through your mind?
>
> P: Well the first that went through my mind was, 'OK, I've got to make Psy' [popular rock star]. Gotta find out what he looks like, 'cause for this I really had no idea, so I started drawing until I was happy with something. Drawing is something I always found fun. So, here he is (pointing to the puppet). I just drew him buff, gave him a batman [costume].
>
> Int: Why did, why did you make him buff?
>
> P: Well he's Batman, he's got to be buff.
>
> Int: Ok, I didn't know that ... What does buff mean to you?
>
> P: Big, muscley [sic], sort of tall.

In this segment, we see a concrete example of the appeal of overt masculinity in this particular boy's description of two male figures in popular media as promoted by the puppets he created. The interviewer's question about the word *buff* and the boy's somewhat exasperated reply ("he's got to be buff") demonstrates language use by adolescents specifically to describe a stereotypical male as "big, muscley, sort of tall."

Later, in response to the interviewer's question about the influence of commercial media on health choices, this same boy engages in far more critical analysis of the interaction between gender and the media and subsequent negative media influences on girls' self-esteem and health choices:

> Int: What about adolescents, kids your age, and younger and a little older? … Is the media giving unhealthy messages? Do you think?
>
> P: … I guess some people could take GI Joes the wrong way or Barbies the wrong way.
>
> P: … I know something from the old Barbie; they apparently used to have like almost an hourglass [figure] or maybe even bigger out here and then here and even shorter through here (gestures to breasts, hips, and waist).
>
> Int: Tiny waist.
>
> P: Like, really tiny waists, super large hips and chest area. They were portrayed as being, like I don't know just.... Not as much nowadays, still they sort of make girls go like, [in a funny voice] 'When I grow up I'm going to get implants!'

Int: So that's a very, that's a definite health hazard that you're noticing.

P: Or like, [funny voice] 'I want to be like Barbie when I grow up!' And then not feeling good about their body. 'I'm going to go get implants!' That's, I guess that's how the implant companies make money.

In this example, dialogue with the interviewer by this point seems to have helped the participant begin to think critically about the power of marketing and to comprehend its relevance in young people's lives (Begoray, Banister, Wharf Higgins, & Wilmot, 2014), far beyond discussions of Batman's appearance.

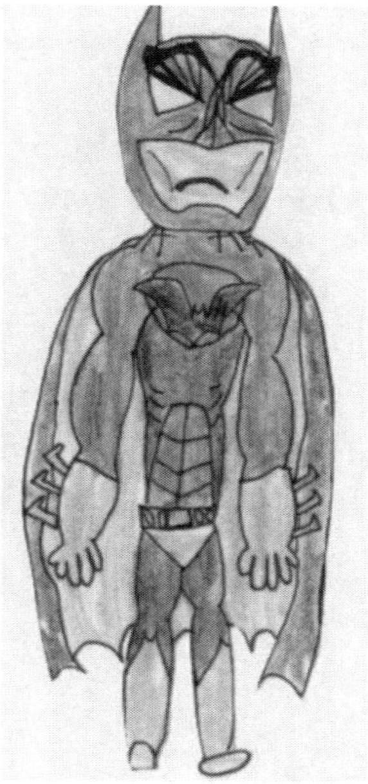

Figure 1. A boy's puppet representing muscular Batman.

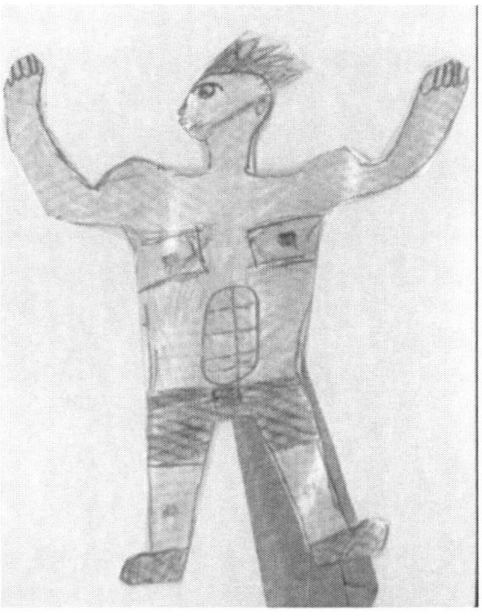

Figure 2. A boy's puppet representing a champion wrestler.

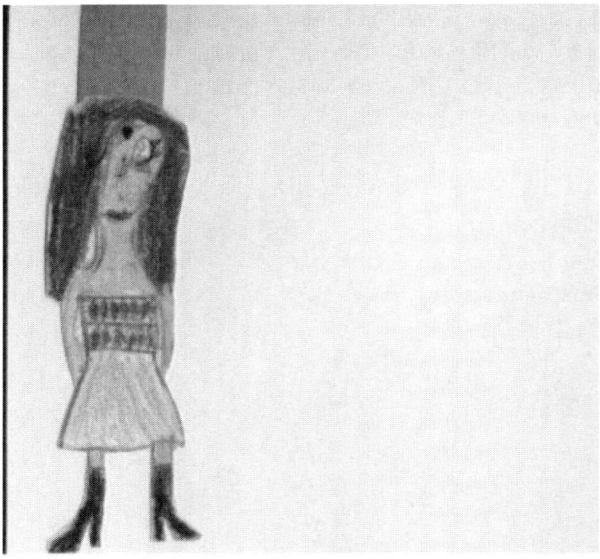

Figure 3. A girl's puppet representing alignment with media stereotypes.

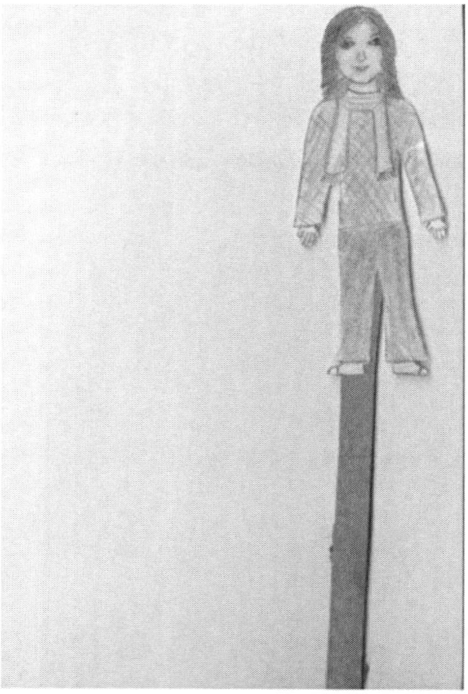

Figure 4. A girl's puppet representing a regular middle school student.

We observed that most but not all of the puppets represented stereotypical physical depictions and expressions of boys/men and girls/women and afforded insight into how participants "perform gender" (Begoray et al., 2015). As we see in the above interview excerpt, puppets created by the boys in general were muscular male figures.

Illustrating the male puppet as muscular "is viewed as a crucial resource for successful performances of masculinity" (MacLean et al., 2010, p. 598). The contrasts in puppets by boys and girls show interesting differences in gender representation. While there were certainly mostly stereotypical puppets (i.e., girls who are dressed like popular singers and boys looking like champion wrestlers), there were also figures more like regular middle school students in t-shirts and pants and an athletic figure looking realistically fit (see Figures 1, 2, 3, & 4).

Individual interviews elicited information without peer pressure and with less likelihood of self-censoring according to traditional notions of femininity and masculinity (Maclean et al., 2010). We also wanted to hear what data focus groups might offer in a more *public* space with a mix of grades and ages but with gender-specific composition.

Focus Groups

Data from seven gender-specific focus groups helped us to gain insight into how gender and media influences were represented in participants' advertisements and, once again, how they used puppets as avatars to represent themselves. Although the students all attended the same middle school, many were not known to each other (e.g., some were enrolled in French immersion and others were regular stream students). The groups that were formed to complete the advertisements were assigned by the classroom teacher to cut across grades and minimize problems. Thus, the result was not natural groups of adolescents who had close affinities (Hyde, Howlett, Brady, & Drennan, 2005); however, they did have 12 hours of working together. We interviewed three groups of girls and four groups of boys, ranging in size from two to five. Small-group size contributes to relatively equal talk time among participants (Raby, 2010). Morgan, Gibbs, Maxwell, and Britten (2002) suggested that focus groups with youth be kept short and that interviewers integrate concrete activities into the discussion. We kept to a maximum 20-minute time schedule for each focus group and included the task of comparing and contrasting class members' puppets.

We also kept field notes of our observations of interactions within each group. Insights into the topic under study can be obtained not only through participants' verbal responses to questions but also by observing the dynamics and responses as members interact with each other. Such social dynamics and actions are "mediated by cultural norms" (Hyde et al., 2005, p. 2593), such as those related to gender.

As with the individual interviews, in order to foster consistency of topics discussed across interviews, we used an interview guide (Appendix B) that included critical questions related to the study. Questions to encourage critical thinking were then posed to foster students' ability to "create, analyse, or evaluate" (Rogow, 2011, p. 19) how gender and the media may have influenced their health advertisements.

Encouraging critical dialogue was sometimes as direct as inquiring about how a gender-specific group's advertisement may have been created differently for an audience of the opposite sex. In the following discussion with a group of boys, this kind of question encouraged some analysis by these boys of how boys and girls are targeted by advertisers:

> Int: What would you have done differently to target girls? To have girls really interested?
>
> P1: I like look at the differences between like boy ads that are more directed towards boys than directed to girls because it is interesting, like if they show the same like toy but they made the girls more pink and the boys like blue and flames, I think it would have

like more, like if it had a girly commercial, if it had like a commercial for girls but it was like a boy toy.

P1: I think girls would still buy it because it showed girls playing with it.

Int: Yah

P2: Yup

P1: and if they saw like boys playing with like a Barbie but they were boys and it was like flames and stuff in the background and it looked like something a boy would do.

P2: Like action figures.

The conversation begins with participants contrasting boys' and girls' toys using stereotypical gender-specific language to describe the toys' clothing as pink or blue. We then see some flexibility away from strict gender categories by these boys with mention that boys can play with boy Barbie dolls (albeit with clothing that is blue). As young people move through adolescence, they become increasingly more sophisticated with their notions of gender and show more fluidity and flexibility in the way they view differences within and similarities between categories of male and female (Martin & Ruble, 2004; Montgomery, 2005). The interviewer's question seemed to foster participants' critical thinking about how advertising works while at the same time revealed a lack of understanding about stereotypical boy and girl behaviours.

Other groups were more readily able to challenge each other's gendered comments to "validate or invalidate their positions" (Hyde et al., 2005, p. 2595), showing more evidence of critical thinking than the group above:

Int: So if you were going to redo this and target it for girls, the girl's team, to make it, because you said it wasn't as popular. What might you have done differently with your ad?

P1: If we were trying to make it for girls only...

P2: We'd probably be like, 'Rugby is awesome.'

P1: And we'd have [rock star] Justin Bieber or One Direction or something come up and say 'Rugby is awesome, now I'm going to sing an annoying song.'

P2: Well, not really like that!

P1: Well, yeah, not like, that 'we're going to sing an annoying song about rugby'. Sorry, that's just my impression of One Direction, and here's my Justin Bieber impression, 'Oh I'm going to sing an annoying song.' That's what I think of them.

Int: Tell me what you were going to say if you were going to retarget this for girls.

P3: If I was going to retarget this, I would probably make it, like, make a fake Justin Bieber and like, play like some sort of song that he sings or something.

[someone singing in the background]

Int: Keep going.

P3: Or like, and then I'd make them say like, 'Rugby is awesome, join [the school] rugby.'

In this conversation, we notice boys' "ritualized forms of humour" (MacLean et al., 2010, p. 598) as a way to help regulate masculinities and construction of hierarchies. The boys appear to be showing off for each other, offering a performance of their identity that not only resembles performances in their everyday culture but also "enables them to sustain a place in the hierarchy of masculinity" (Hyde et al., 2005, p. 2593). Social dynamics in an interview setting are "mediated by cultural norms [and in this instance capture] a central feature of male youth culture" (Hyde et al., 2005, p. 2593). Nevertheless, despite the boys' lightheartedness, the notion of girls joining the rugby team was acknowledged. In addition, Participant 2 challenged Participant 1's description of including Justin Bieber to target their advertisement to an audience of girls. In response to the challenge, the participant apologized and justified his original idea of using Justin Bieber. This exchange follows with Participant 3 supporting the idea of using the teen rock star along with some music (while in the background Participant 1 is singing a Justin Bieber song).

Earlier in the research study when this group was formulating ideas for their advertisement, we observed that one boy's suggestion to include representations of girls in the ad was adamantly shut down by another and more dominant group member. Morrow (2006) pointed out that middle adolescents tend to demonstrate rigid, stereotypical understandings of gender differences and that their expectations of how their peers should behave can reinforce gender stereotypes.

The following focus group with girls illustrates many stereotypical views about gender expectations and roles for boys and girls:

> Int: If you were trying to attract boys, more boys to leadership, how would you have shaped your advertisement differently?
>
> P3: We probably would have added…
>
> P5: [interruption] Gangnam Style! [a song popular with boys in this class]
>
> [Laughter]
>
> P4: Or we probably would have added in more of the athletic leadership. Because with the athletic leadership that we have here it's, what is it? You two (gesturing to two other group members) are in leadership now.
>
> P5: Adding in the jobs that are like, guys would more likely do.
>
> P1: So like the Terry Fox run.
>
> P5: I think girls like, no, guys like running that. Girls like more organizing things and then boys don't-
>
> P3: Yah.
>
> P4: They just sort of go along with it and help us a lot.
>
> P1: I don't want to be stereotypical but I think boys are not as focused on being organized and they just want to have fun with some things, so that's why our [ad] was, it wasn't like some of the boys' [ads] that had a lot of kind of funny parts to it and funny jokes in there. Ours was more reasons why it was a good idea to join, and I think...
>
> P5: It was more, like, educational.
>
> P1: Yah, I think.
>
> P3: If you tried to kind of turn it to our, try to involve boys as well, it would have been a little more, it would have been more kind of … maybe goofy's not the best word, but kind of a little more jokes and more fun with it and so.
>
> P2: Well, we're having fun with it.

When asked about their advertisement on leadership and how this could be adapted differently to attract boys, the girls identified that they would need a more athletic focus, include the rock star Psy (whose song Gangnam Style was popular at the time of this research and used in a boy's advertisement described above), use jokes, be goofy, and have more fun. They observed that, in comparison with the boys' advertisements that were filled with funny jokes, their advertisement was educational. Participant 1 said that she did not want to be stereotypical but that girls are more organized and focused than boys in terms of leadership tasks, such as organizing a Terry Fox run. They are aware of the stereotypes used on the opposite gender. However, a comment that resists gender stereotyping emerged when Participant 2 asserts that they too are having fun with their advertisement.

Overall, focus groups showed what girls and boys thought about gendered behaviours in their day-to-day school experiences as well as in advertisements. Their small-group interactions revealed their stance toward gender. These beliefs and behaviours would be appropriate topics of lessons in all adolescent health education classes.

Health Education Implications

Health education programs vary considerably; however, in BC there is a need to open space in schools for critical dialogue and reflection related to gender and interaction with health-related media messages. For example, the BC Physical and Health Education, Grade 8 curriculum (MOE, 2013b) refers to *gender* only once. While *communication* remains a core competency (i.e., a general ability that permeates all subject areas), a teacher in BC would need to work in an interdisciplinary fashion with the English Language Arts curriculum (MOE, 2013a) to search for competencies that address the skill of critical thinking. There is, however, no specific reference to this competency. The English Language Arts curriculum does state that "students will be able to develop and defend a position with supporting evidence" (MOE, 2013a, n.p.).

Health educators might be advised to use literacy concepts combined with health concepts on gender to help students become more health literate. While teaching examples are promised in these draft documents, at this writing there are no specific ideas for teachers to follow on the development of critical thinking around gender in the health education classroom. Our study demonstrates one potential approach to meeting this goal by engaging students in a hands-on creative project and by fostering critical thinking through reflection. While our emphasis in this study was on research, these approaches are valid for pedagogy in middle years' classrooms.

Methodological Implications

Our methods in this study suggest their use is appropriate for other investigations with adolescents; for example, in lessons that allow for in-process interaction with students and our approach to individual interviews and focus groups. The context of our study offered a window to observe how gender and sex is "implicit and performative" (Haines et al., 2009, p. 2035). We observed behaviours during the lessons and were able to talk with students because they were engaged in student-centered, small-group projects, rather than being in more teacher-centered lectures. Student-based classes were the norm at this school, and we were able to further decenter activities by providing technical assistance to each group in the form of a graduate student helper. Possibilities emerged not only for performance but also for some participants to pose ideas that went against group norms (Hyde et al., 2005).

Throughout the study, participants revealed their understanding of gendered messages as we sought their ideas while they were doing classroom work as well as following up with more conventional focus groups.

We noticed that participants enacted different aspects of their identities in the social and media contexts within which they were engaged (Pink, 2001). They appeared to be concerned with producing public impressions (MacLean et al., 2010) of how their puppets represented gender. For example, their puppet creations served to visually represent their embodied performances of gender identities and illustrate their views of masculinity and femininity.

Interviews featured questions to foster critical thinking and reflection by students. As previously discussed, questions that were authentic conversation openers and had no specific answer resulted in students' voices and opinions being a focus of our study. Using concrete objects (i.e., the puppets they created) as one impetus for conversation gave further focus to adolescents who sometimes need such props to foster more abstract thinking. Irvin and Strauss (2000) commented that "guided discussion help[s] students learn social skills ... receive validation for their ideas and opinions and have the opportunity to consider the viewpoints of others ... understand, internalize and benefit from new insights" (p. 120). Our interviews showed these adolescents engaged in authentic discussion.

Suggestions for Future Research

Our methods can be applied to other research with adolescents. Consideration of biological–developmental stages of adolescents is important to remember; however, equally important, adolescents are individuals shaped by the social context of our consumer society. Bottorff et al. (2012) argued that, in any research on men's and women's or girls' and boys' health, qualitative researchers address how and whether gender (or sociocultural considerations) are accounted for and how "biological (sex) factors may be interacting with gender and should be explored" (p. 438). Within this classroom of students in Grades 6–8, there were tall boys with shadows of facial hair and small boys with smooth-faces; there were girls with breasts and hips and girls without. Researchers might look at how gender conceptions of adolescents vary before and after reaching puberty.

Further work must be done on a variety of gender messages beyond those of advertisers to more general ones in other media such as those embedded in regular television programming. How do stars of popular programs play out stereotypical gender roles? How do they challenge gender roles? What are the common stereotypes surrounding adolescents as a group or as male and female teens? How might students themselves discover these stereotypes and challenge them?

Limitations

Despite our efforts to create an authentic and valid investigation, our study inevitably had limitations. The main limitation was in our conceptualization of *gender*. Universal characteristics cannot be generalized to all boys and girls (Morrow, 2006). Research needs to move "beyond the binary," and we acknowledge that we have relied too heavily on "conceptually stagnant notions of gender and sex that contrast masculine males with feminine females" (Johnson & Repta, 2010, p. 17) which serves to only "reinstate gender binaries" Haines et al., 2009, p. 2036). Nevertheless, we believe that our study presents valuable findings about the ability of some young adolescents to grapple with stereotypical gender norms established and aggressively maintained by advertisers.

We did not collect data about how the gender of researchers and research assistants may have influenced relations with participants. All researchers were women and only two of the graduate student research assistants were men. Participants did not have any choice about the research assistant assigned to each group in terms of gender nor did we offer any choice to research assistants.

Finally, we recognize that we need to further modify our interviewing techniques with adolescents to obtain even more valid data. "Interview talk" (Abell, Locke, Condor, Gibson, & Stevenson, 2006, p. 230), that is, researchers' language use and questions, can influence adolescent participants' responses and information they disclose. We might, for example, move to even less-structured interviews to elicit more genuine conversation and have prompts reviewed by middle years' teachers to ask for further suggestions about language.

Conclusion

Our study gave adolescent participants an active role in creating knowledge about the topic of inquiry (Gomez, Puigvert, & Flecha, 2011), in this case, an advertisement for a healthy activity. We provided an opportunity for these adolescents to demonstrate how they were "active agents in their construction of gender" (MacLean et al., 2010, p. 598).

We observed the ways in which the adolescents performed gender, how their social context offered a segue into understanding the link between our "localized observations and broader macro-level structures (Chabot & Shoveller, 2012, p. 122), and how, for example, norms of adolescent masculinity and femininity reaffirm the "heteronormativity of the school culture" (Haines et al., 2009, p. 2030). Their largely stereotypical thinking is not surprising, given advertisers' sophistication with targeting young people based on gender and age (Buckingham as cited in Morrow, 2006), which they modeled in their own advertisements, and the gendered patterns of mid adolescents' culture.

Caldwell (2012) commented that "gender stereotypes can limit [adolescents'] individuality, compromise their integrity and affect their self-esteem" (p. 10). Our study shows that some adolescents demonstrated more flexibility than Morrow (2006) suggested, however, and were occasionally able to challenge conceptions; for example, when a girl commented that her group is having fun even though other girls in her group had attributed fun as a concern for boys. In addition, both girls and boys showed some understanding of how the opposite gender is stereotyped. They were able to suggest how their own ads could be modified to appeal to an audience of the opposite gender. These changes were, however, largely stereotypical in content.

In conclusion, we maintain that developing a greater understanding of the influence of gender on adolescent health will afford the development of gender-appropriate interventions that can serve to help improve health education, improve adolescent health literacy, and empower researchers to investigate adolescent health literacy more effectively.

Questions for Discussion, Reflection, and Writing

1. How can critical questions be used to help students challenge gendered health messages in media advertising?
2. What kinds of concrete activities can educators use to help adolescents discuss abstract concepts such as gender?
3. Why is personal experience of adolescents relevant in adolescent learning about gender and health?

List of Online Resources

- Canadian Institutes of Health Research: Institute of Gender and Health – http://www.cihr-irsc.gc.ca/e/8673.html
- Media Smarts: Canada's Centre for Digital and Media Literacy Marketing to Teens: Gender Roles in Advertising – Lesson – http://mediasmarts.ca/lessonplan/marketing-teens-gender-roles-advertising-lesson

Appendix A. Interview Guide for Individuals

1. Tell me about your puppet (probe for details of dress, makeup, muscles, etc.).
2. Show participant the group of boy puppets and group of girl puppets created by others. What details do you notice? What are the differences between the girl and boy puppets? In what way might you see the same thing in professional ads?
3. What do you think (opposite gender) would say about your puppet? Why?
4. How might you see the role of girls (or boys) differently in professional ads as a result of creating your puppet?

Appendix B. Interview Guide for Focus Groups

1. Describe your ad for me and how you decided on the topic – especially since we are talking about media and health.
2. How did you decide to use girls *(or boys or both)* for your audience in ads that are promoting healthy living activities?
3. At the very beginning of our time at *(the school)*, the group was asked to describe how advertisers "hook" people. There were lots of interesting ideas. How and why might advertisers use different strategies to hook boys than they do to hook girls?
4. Tell me about how you used advertising strategies to "hook" *(the school)* girls *(or boys or both)* to sign up for your activity? What skills did you or someone in your group already have that you used to create this ad?
5. What would you do differently if you were creating this ad for *(boys or girls)*?
6. How were your sets and/or puppets created so that you could hook boys or girls or both? What about your puppets' actions and the script?

7. How did being a *(boy or girl)* influence the way you created your set, script, puppets?
8. What did you learn about targeting boys or girls during this project?
9. Thinking about what you know about how advertisers target adolescent girls and boys, how would you question ads that you saw on television or the computer or in magazines now? *(ask for an example)*.
10. What do you think about using advertising strategies deliberately to hook *(your school's)* students?

References

Abell, J., Locke, A., Condor, S., Gibson, S., & Stevenson, C. (2006). Trying similarity, doing difference: The role of interviewer self-disclosure in interview talk with young people. *Qualitative Research, 6*(2), 221–244.

Archer, L. (2002). "It's easier that you're a girl and that you're Asian": Interactions of 'race' and gender between researchers and participants. *Feminist Review, 72*(1), 108–132.

Ashcraft, C. (2012). But how do we talk about it? Critinal literacy practices for addressing sexuality with youth. *Curriculum Inquiry, 42*(5), 597–628.

Banister, E., Begoray, D., & Daly, K. (2011). Responding to adolescent women's reproductive health concerns: Empowering clients through health literacy. *Health Care for Women International, 32*(4), 344–354.

Begoray, D., Banister, E., Wharf Higgins, J., & Wilmot, R. (2014). Online, tuned in, turned on: Multimedia approaches to fostering critical media health literacy for adolescents. *Asia-Pacific Journal of Health, Sport and Physical Education, 5*(3), 267-280.

Begoray, D., Banister, E., Wharf Higgins, J., & Wilmot, R. (2015). Puppets on a string? How young adolescents explore gender and health in advertising. *Journal of Media Literacy Education, 6*(3), 57–64.

Begoray, D., Wharf Higgins, J., Harrison, J., & Collins-Emery, A. (2013). Adolescent reading/viewing of advertisements: Understandings from transactional and positioning theory. *Journal of Adolescent & Adult Literacy, 57*(2), 121–130.

Begoray, D., Wharf Higgins, J., & MacDonald, M. (2009). High school health curriculum and health literacy: Canadian student voices. *Global Health Promotion, 16*(4), 34–42.

Bergsma, L. (2011). Media literacy and health promotion for adolescents. *Journal of Media Literacy Education*, 3(1), Article 10. Retrieved from http://digitalcommons.uri.edu/jmle/vol3/iss1/10

Bottorff, J. L., Oliffe, J. L., & Kelly, M. T. (2012). The gender(s) in the room. *Qualitative Health Research, 22*(4), 435–440.

Bottorff, J. L., Oliffe, J. L., Kelly, M. T., & Chambers, N. A. (2011). Approaches to examining gender relations in health research. In J. L. Oliffe & L. Greaves (Eds.), *Designing and conducting gender, sex, health research* (pp. 175–188). Thousand Oaks, CA: SAGE.

British Columbia Ministry of Education. (2013a). *English language arts, grade 8*. Victoria, BC: Author. Retrieved from https://curriculum.gov.bc.ca/curriculum/English%20Language%20Arts/8

British Columbia Ministry of Education. (2013b). *Physical and health education, grade 8.* Victoria, BC: Author. Retrieved from https://curriculum.gov.bc.ca/curriculum/Physical%20and%20Health%20Education/8

Caldwell, M. (2012). Inquiry into identity: Teaching critical thinking through race, class and gender. *Middle School Journal, 43*(4), 6–15.

Chabot, C., & Shoveller, J. (2012). Fieldwork: Observations and interviews. In J. L. Oliffe & L. Greaves (Eds.), *Designing and conducting gender, sex, health research* (pp. 105–126). Thousand Oaks, CA: SAGE.

Facione, P. A. (1990). *Critical thinking: A statement of expert consensus for purposes of educational assessment and instruction* (Executive Summary). Milbrae, CA: California Academic Press. Retrieved from http://assessment.aas.duke.edu/documents/Delphi_Report.pdf

Flecha, A., Pulido, C., & Christou, M. (2011). Transforming violent selves through reflection in critical communicative research. *Qualitative Inquiry, 17*(3), 246–255.

Gómez, A., Puigvert, L., & Flecha, R. (2011). Critical communicative methodology: Informing real social transformation through research. *Qualitative Inquiry, 17*(3), 235–245.

Haines, R. J., Johnson, J. L., Carter, C. I., & Arora, K. (2009). "I couldn't say, I'm not a girl": Adolescents talk about gender and marijuana use. *Social Science & Medicine, 68*(11), 2029–2036.

Hyde, A., Howlett, E., Brady, D., & Drennan, J. (2005). The focus group method: Insights from focus group interviews on sexual health with adolescents. *Social Science & Medicine, 61*(12), 2588–2599.

Irvin, J., & Strauss, S. (2000). Developmental tasks of early adolescence. In K. Woods & T. Dickinson (Eds.), *Promoting literacy in grades 4–9* (pp. 115–127). Boston, MA: Allyn & Bacon.

Jeong, S-H., Cho, H., & Hwang, Y. (2012). Media literacy interventions: A meta-analytic review. *Journal of Communication, 62*(3), 454–472.

Johnson, J. L., & Repta, R. (2012). Sex and gender: Beyond the binaries. In J. L. Oliffe & L. Greaves (Eds.), *Designing and conducting gender, sex, health research* (pp. 17–37). Thousand Oaks, CA: SAGE.

MacLean, A., Sweeting, H., & Hunt, K. (2010). 'Rules' for boys, 'guidelines' for girls: Gender differences in symptom reporting during childhood and adolescence. *Social Science & Medicine, 70*(4), 597–604.

Manago, A. M., Graham, M. B., Greenfield, P. M., & Salimkhan, G. (2008). Self-presentation and gender on MySpace. *Journal of Applied Developmental Psychology, 29*(6), 446–458.

Martin, C. L., & Ruble, D. (2004). Children's search for gender cues: Cognitive perspectives on gender development. *Current Directions in Psychological Science, 13*(2), 67–70.

Montgomery, M. J. (2005). Psychosocial intimacy and identity: From early adolescence to emerging adulthood. *Journal of Adolescent Research, 20*(3), 346–374.

Morgan, M., Gibbs, S., Maxwell, K., & Britten, N. (2002). Hearing children's voices: Methodological issues in conducting focus groups with children aged 7–11 years. *Qualitative Research, 2*(5), 5–20.

Morrow, V. (2006). Understanding gender differences in context: Implications for young children's everyday lives. *Children & Society, 20*(2), 92–104.

Oliver, K. (2001). Images of the body from popular culture: Engaging adolescent girls in critical inquiry. *Sports, Education and Society, 6*(2), 143–164.

Pink, S. (2001). More visualising, more methodologies: On video, reflexivity and qualitative research. *Sociological Review*, *49*(4), 586–599.

Raby, R. (2010). Public selves, inequality, and interruptions: The creation of meaning in focus groups with teens. *International Journal of Qualitative Methods, 9*(1), 1–16.

Rogow, F. (2011). Ask, don't tell: Pedagogy for media literacy education in the next decade. *Journal of Media Literacy Education*, *3*(1), 16–22.

Scull, T. M., Malik, C.V., & Kupersmidt, J. B. (2014). A media literacy education approach to teaching adolescents comprehensive sexual health education. *Journal of Media Literacy Education*, *6*(1), 1–14.

ter Bogt, T., Engels, R., Bogers, S., & Kloosterman, M. (2010). "Shake it baby, shake it": Media preferences, sexual attitudes and gender stereotypes among adolescents. *Sex Roles*, *63*, 844–859.

Weaver, C., & Alvermann, D. E. (2000). Critical thinking and discussion. In K. Wood & T. Dickinson (Eds.), *Promoting literacy in grades 4–9: A handbook for teachers and administrators* (pp. 344–351. Boston, MA: Allyn & Bacon.

Wolsey, T., & Lapp, D. (2009). Discussion-based instruction in the middle and secondary school classroom. In K. Wood & W. Blanton, *Literacy instruction for adolescents: Research based practice* (pp. 368–391). New York, NY: Guilford Press.

Yin, R. K. (2009). *Case study research: Design and methods* (4th ed.). Thousand Oaks, CA: SAGE.

In: Adolescent Health Literacy and Learning
Editors: D. L. Begoray and E. M. Banister
ISBN: 978-1-63482-897-0

Chapter 6

FAST FOOD VS. FITNESS: GENDERED HEALTH LITERACY NEEDS OF SECONDARY SCHOOL STUDENTS

Joan Wharf Higgins* and Kai Bellows Riecken
School of Exercise Science, Physical & Health Education,
University of Victoria, Canada

ABSTRACT

Embedded in a comprehensive school health model, this chapter describes a study that sought to engage students both within and beyond the classroom to improve their health behaviours. We recount our experiences investigating the health practices of secondary school students (N = 441) in British Columbia, Canada, including a gendered analysis of their self-reported physical activity, healthy eating and sedentary behaviours, and accelerometers to objectively measure physical activity. Students completed additional questionnaires to measure intrinsic and extrinsic motivations for being physically active and eating healthfully. Students' height, weight, and body circumference were also assessed. Finally, focus groups captured their perspectives of engaging in health practices qualitatively. We found students were far from meeting national recommendations for fruit and vegetable consumption, screen time, and sugar-sweetened beverage intake and for moderate-to-vigorous physical activity (as measured by accelerometry). Moreover, the data revealed some gendered differences: boys were found have both higher physical activity levels and intrinsic motivation scores to be active, while girls exhibited healthier eating patterns and a greater motivation for doing so. There were no differences in male and female students' sedentary practices. Interpreted though a definition of health literacy, focus group data revealed students' insights into accessing, understanding, evaluating, and communicating health information. Using a health literacy lens to interpret these findings, we argue that secondary curricula need to accommodate the gendered nature of youth health literacy needs. At the same time, a deeper understanding of the specifics of youth sedentary practices can contribute to a more gender-inclusive curriculum.

* Correspondence to (email): jwharfhi@uvic.ca

Keywords: physical activity, healthy eating, health literacy, gender, comprehensive school health

INTRODUCTION

Focusing Questions

1. Think back to when you were in secondary school: was there a difference between the health practices of boys and girls? If so, what were these differences?
2. What about being in secondary school might contribute to girls and boys sharing and/or differing in their health practices?

Because the majority of adolescents spend a substantial amount of time in a common setting, the secondary school setting represents, for many, the last cost-free opportunity to learn about health and develop healthy living practices. No other institution has as much continuous and intensive contact with youth during the adolescent years (Story, Kaphingst, & French, 2006). Moreover, schools can help to address health inequities as they reach adolescents from diverse race and socioeconomic backgrounds (Kriemler et al., 2011), providing fair distribution of resources during the time they are on campus (Institute of Medicine & National Research Council, 2009). Thus, schools have an unparalleled — and perhaps the only — opportunity to impact the health of youth; they have been identified by researchers for over a decade as a critical setting for intervention (Raine, 2004). In this chapter, we describe our experience with the health-promoting secondary schools (HPSS) initiative in 10 British Columbia (BC) secondary schools. The HPSS research study sought to enhance the physical activity/sedentary and eating practices of Grade 10 students through the physical education (PE) and health education curricula as well as school-wide policies and culture. Our results are discussed in terms of health literacy concepts and offer a gendered perspective on the health literacy needs of secondary school students. In the literature, gender is regarded as one of the individual characteristics or traits — along with race, socioeconomic status, culture, language, education, and cognitive and social skills — that influence adolescent health literacy (Manganello, 2008). Although it is unclear in the literature whether the use of *gender* refers to biological sex alone or a more cultural interpretation of gender as masculine and feminine orientation, we expect that it is the former rather than the latter. The term *adolescent health literacy* is not yet well defined. It is frequently expressed as health-related knowledge (DeWalt & Hink, 2009) but also as an interactive and critical skill set to help youth act in health-enhancing ways: "Those between the ages of 3 and 18 can seek, comprehend, evaluate, and use health information, especially if materials are presented in ways that are age appropriate, culturally relevant, and socially supported" (Borzekowski, 2009, p. S288).

We begin the chapter with brief reviews of youth health and health practices, what is known of the health literacy of adolescents, and then report on the HPSS intervention and methodology of the study. Presentation of the results follow, and the chapter concludes with an interpretation of the results in terms of the gendered health literacy needs of secondary school students.

HEALTH AND HEALTH PRACTICES OF ADOLESCENTS

Adolescence should be a stage in which physical health is not an issue — when the body is young and growing and supports young people in their educational and social pursuits. Only recently has the health care profession been called to tend to health issues usually relegated toward later stages of life such as increasing rates of diabetes, high blood pressure, and other conditions not typically present until adulthood (Gray et al., 2014). Similarly, concern over youths' unhealthy practices contributing to such conditions has been raised by health promotion and education scholars: physical activity (PA) rates decline substantially from childhood to adolescence with 87% of youth failing to attain the recommended 90 minutes of moderate-to-vigorous PA per day (Colley et al., 2011) while they spend at least 3 hours a day watching television or playing video games (Molt, McAuley, Birnbaum, & Lytle, 2006) and several more connected online (Jones & Fox, 2009), consume high amounts of sugar-sweetened beverages (SSB; French, Lin, & Guthrie, 2003), and eat less than the recommended amount of fruits and vegetables (BC Ministry of Health Services, 2004). Sedentary behaviour, in particular, has been linked to higher consumption of SSBs and lower intake of fruits and vegetables (Pearson & Biddle, 2011). Alarmingly, only 8% of Canadian youth aged 12–17 were found to engage in all three *asset behaviours* — achieving the recommended activity level, engaging in 2 hours or less of screen time, and consuming 5 or more servings of fruits and vegetables (Canadian Institute for Health Information, 2009).

Collectively, low levels of PA, high levels of sedentary behaviour, and unhealthy eating habits may substantially affect the prevalence of cancers, diabetes, and other chronic diseases into the future (American Cancer Society, 2008). Concurrent with this rise in health problems, hours devoted to health education curricula in BC secondary schools have dwindled over the past 10 years, resulting in only 20% of Grade 12 students indicating they were learning how to stay healthy at school (BC Office of the Provincial Health Officer, 2008). Thus brews the perfect storm: more sedentary and fewer physical activity behaviours, increased consumption of low nutrition/calorically dense foods, and a decreased role for schools in providing PA and health education opportunities.

Gendered Health Practices

Male and female youths exhibit similar levels of sedentary behaviours (Pearson & Biddle, 2011) but differ in their PA and eating patterns. Adolescents' fondness for *screens* seems to be gender neutral with both boys and girls engaged for multiple hours each day with their phones, playing video games, watching television, and using computers for recreational networking and enjoyment (Pujazon-Zazik & Park, 2010).

We have known for many years that boys are more physically active than girls (Coombes, Jones, Page, & Cooper, 2014; Wharf Higgins, Gaul, Gibbons, & Van Gyn, 2003) and, although closing, this gap remains today (Tremblay et al., 2010). Youths' perceived competence to perform activities and its influence on their sense of enjoyment have been shown to be important factors influencing youths' participation in physical activity, especially for girls as they age (Cairney et al., 2012).

The recent implementation of female-tailored and female-only PE classes in BC and Canada — emphasizing participation over performance and a wide variety of activities rather than just sports — has served to somewhat mitigate this disparity (Gibbons, 2014).

Gender differences in dietary knowledge, affect, and behaviours have been established (Orji, Vassileva, & Mandryk, 2013), leading to calls for gender-specific interventions to address the different motivations for the eating decisions by males and females. For example, Orji et al. (2013) found females to be more knowledgeable about nutrition and driven by more holistic and realistic perceptions of healthy eating (e.g., concern for disease, healthy weight) while males were less concerned with the impact of diet on disease and indulged in more fast food meals. Others have found female students to consume fewer soft drinks than male students while a higher intake of fruits and vegetables was more related to family income than gender (Rovner, Nansel, Wang, & Iannotti, 2011).

Health Literacy of Adolescents

The clinical and health-promoting concepts of health literacy are often measured in adults, particularly in relationship to use of health services and health outcomes. However, the application and measurement of health literacy among youth is less well understood (Manganello, 2008) largely due to the lack of an agreed-upon operational definition and adequate, accurate measurement tools (Ormshaw, Paakkari, & Kannas, 2013; Perry, 2014). With the exception of the work by Wu et al. (2010) and Levin-Zamir, Lemish, and Gofin (2011), the few tools that exist for adolescents measure limited aspects of health literacy such as reading ability (Davis, Wolf, Bass et al., 2006) and self-reported health literacy (Norman & Skinner, 2006) or are limited to screening youths' health literacy (e.g., Rapid Assessment of Adolescent Literacy in Medicine–Teen; Davis, Wolf, Arnold et al., 2006) in a health-care context (Massey et al., 2013). This dearth of metrics and evidence of adolescents' health literacy should not be taken as a lack of importance; achieving health literacy is a necessary step on the way to healthy behaviour (Deaton, 2002). Ormshaw et al. (2013) stated, "health literacy, as an outcome, or result of education and training, can clearly be seen as a prerequisite or mediating factor for the creation and motivation of the empowered individual" (p. 434).

Research results suggest that low health literacy rates among youth is connected to risky behaviours (Conwell et al., 2003), obesity (Chari, Warsh, Ketterer, Hossain, & Sharif, 2014), and less health-promoting behaviour (Chang, 2011). Moreover, health literacy for adolescents is viewed as a necessary life skill to negotiate the complex demands of modern society (Kickbusch & Maag, 2008) and as an element of citizenship (Paakkari & Paakkari, 2012; Sorenson et al., 2012).

That health literacy is so strongly, but not always clearly, tied to healthy behaviours and outcomes explains why it has joined the long list of factors delineating what makes people healthy. As Simonds (1974) suggested four decades ago and echoed by St. Leger (2001) in the last decade and by Marks and Wharf Higgins (2012) in the current decade, schools offer the setting and opportunities to nurture a health-literate constituency.

Health-Promoting Secondary Schools

Health promotion and education in the secondary school setting may be one effective vehicle to reverse negative health trends and enhance health literacy. Given the layered and connected influences within secondary schools (Deschesnes, Martin, & Jomphe Hill, 2003), a health curriculum alone may be insufficient to facilitate healthy living among youth (Naylor, Macdonald, Warburton, Reed, & McKay, 2008).

Thus, comprehensive school health models that address the many layers and multiple influences have garnered increased attention and have been cited as one of the seven best investments to address the worldwide physical inactivity crisis (Blanchard, Shilton, & Bull, 2013; Kohl et al., 2012).

To date, such models have been implemented largely within elementary and middle schools (Stone, McKenzie, Welk, & Booth, 1998), with considerably fewer at the secondary school level.

Based on the urgency of the epidemiological evidence and success of comprehensive school models in addressing students' health, we and our colleagues developed, implemented, and evaluated the HPSS initiative (2010–13) in 10 BC secondary schools. Funded by the Canadian Cancer Society's Prevention Initiative, the overall intent of HPSS was to increase the levels of PA and fruit and vegetable consumption and to decrease the amount of screen time and SSB consumption among youth enrolled in the intervention schools. The study's design and results related to these primary outcomes are described in detail elsewhere (Wharf Higgins et al., 2013, 2014).

Although not specifically designed to address nor measure the health literacy of students, we suggest that the use of the PE and health education curricula and focus on teaching and learning within these classrooms offers a glimpse into health literacy of this sample of Grade 10 students in BC.

The HPSS intervention consisted of four aspects. First, PE 10 and Health 10 classes offered students choice-based learning activities. Within these courses, complete curricula guides were developed with and for teachers and offered detailed lesson plans, handouts, assessment and tracking tools, a calendar for implementing the lessons, and background information related to the target health behaviours. Second, we asked schools to provide opportunities for students to increase their knowledge and abilities outside the classroom through school-wide events and policies. HPSS intervention schools were asked to carry out at least two school-wide events or activities and to make one policy change that best reflected their local needs and interests.

Third, our grant allowed us to directly support teaching and learning. Each intervention school received \$4,100 at the beginning of the school year to either purchase necessary equipment or support professional development, staff, or events including \$2,500 to support infrastructure or environmental changes at the school.

Finally, we asked schools to engage their students in the design and delivery of school-wide events, activities, and policies. Schools were asked to establish an Action Team (6–10 members) with 50% adult and 50% youth participation and to create an Action Plan for their school.

METHODS

Design

The HPSS study was considered a real community trial (Wharf Higgins et al., 2013), merging quasi-experimental and community-based methodologies to meet the needs of each school while maintaining procedural rigour. The Human Research Ethics Boards at both the Universities of Victoria and British Columbia approved the project. Consenting schools (N = 10) were then matched based on demographic and geographic similarity and randomly assigned to a waitlisted control group (n = 5) or the intervention group (n = 5). In September 2011 (T1), quantitative baseline data were collected and the intervention was initiated within the schools. Post-intervention data were collected at the end of the academic year in May and June 2012 (T2). Focus groups were conducted only at T2 with the five intervention schools for the purpose of better understanding the implementation process and stakeholder perspective throughout the project. Due to the influence of a teachers' strike on the implementation of the HPSS intervention and subsequent behavioural results at T2 (Wharf Higgins et al., 2014), in this chapter we use a combination of the quantitative data gathered at T1 from all intervention and control schools and from the focus group data from intervention schools to describe the eating and activity behaviours of these adolescents for discussion within the context of health literacy. Informed consent was obtained from all participants. The results are limited by the reliance on cross-sectional, self-report data with the exception of accelerometry to objectively capture physical activity from a volunteer sample; therefore, we do not assume that our findings are relevant for other students.

Instruments

The Canadian School Health Action, Planning, and Evaluation System (SHAPES) questionnaire, a valid and reliable measure for health behaviours (Biddle, Gorely, Pearson, & Bull, 2011), was used to capture student demographics, self-reported height and weight, physical activity, sedentary behaviours, and healthy eating (HE) behaviours (N = 441). Moderate-to-vigorous PA (MVPA) was based on a 7-day recall of minutes of activity per day. From this total, weekend minutes, weekday minutes, and average minutes per day of MVPA were extrapolated. Sedentary time was also a recall of total time spent on inactive pastimes (e.g., television and Internet surfing) on an average day. MVPA was measured objectively at T1 (N = 270) using ActiGraph GM1 accelerometers (Esliger, Copeland, Barnes, & Tremblay, 2005). Based on current recommendations, accelerometers were worn for seven days and daily log books were submitted (Robertson, Stewart-Brown, Wilcock, Oldfield, & Thorogood, 2011). Using the cut points outlined by Evenson, Catellier, Gill, Ondrak, and McMurray (2008), totals and averages for minutes of weekly, weekend, and weekday MVPA were calculated.

Healthy eating was based on a series of questions in the SHAPES survey pertaining to servings of foods and beverages consumed over the previous 24 hours as well as behaviour pattern queries (e.g., eating breakfast, eating with adults or in front of the television). Questions for fruits and vegetables asked how many half-cup servings, or one-cup servings in the case of leafy greens, of fruits and vegetables were consumed the previous day. For beverages, students were asked to report how many servings of each type of beverage (e.g., one cup, drinking box, one can) were consumed the previous day. Sugary drinks were considered to be all those beverages containing sugar calories from added or natural sources (e.g., soft drink or 100% fruit juice, respectively), while SSBs were defined as those drinks containing added sugars (e.g., energy drinks, 'slurpees'). Finally, students completed a series of established questionnaires, tailored slightly to the context of PE and health education, to assess their intrinsic and extrinsic sources of motivation for PA and HE (Markland & Tobin, 2004).

Focus groups with students included those in PE and Health 10 ($n = 63$) and Action Team members ($n = 34$) were conducted to gather their perspectives regarding their experience with HPSS overall. Open-ended questions related to the health behaviours of interest were posed by a trained interviewer. The focus groups were audio recorded and notes were taken.

Data Analyses

Quantitative data were analyzed in SPSS 22.0. Those with missing data for a given outcome variable were not included in the related analysis. For the purposes of this chapter, questions relevant to health literacy or relevant health behaviours (e.g., physical activity, healthy eating, sedentary time) were analyzed for basic descriptive data, correlations, and *t*-tests by gender to examine any trends that may have occurred. ActiGraph data were processed using KineSoft© (http://www.kinesoft.org) to tabulate MVPA minutes. Accelerometer data analysis was based on 15-second epochs and PA intensity level cut points were based on validated recommendations in the literature (Evenson et al., 2008). Only those students with a minimum of three valid weekdays and one valid weekend day (10 or more hours of wear time) were used in subsequent analyses.

Verbatim transcriptions for all focus groups were completed and subsequently analysed in NVivo™ 10.0 (http://www.qsrinternational.com). In cases where audio files were inaudible or otherwise unusable, facilitator notes were transcribed. Open coding of the focus groups was used to classify data into potential categories and themes (Patton, 2002). During this process of open coding, any quotations related to the central components of health literacy (i.e., access, understand, evaluate, communicate) (Rootman & Gordon-El-Bihbety, 2008) were coded as such. A second round of coding identified subthemes related to health literacy content. These data were not separated by gender as the focus groups were a mix of males and females; however, comments that specifically mentioned gender differences were sequestered for this chapter.

RESULTS

Students had a median age of 15.3 years at T1 and a median body mass index (BMI) of 21.9, which is within the healthy BMI range for their age. There were comparable numbers of male (50.3%) and female (49.7%) students involved, most of whom self-identified as Caucasian (67%) and who stated an average household income of $80,097 (Wharf Higgins et al., 2013; n.b., the SHAPES questionnaire asked students to self-identify only as male or female).

Survey Results

The data collected from the student surveys highlight several interesting behavioural trends. As presented in Table 1, students were far from meeting national recommendations for fruit and vegetable consumption, screen time, and SSB intake and for MVPA (as measured by accelerometry). As measured by both SHAPES and accelerometry, on average boys were more active than girls on weekdays and weekends but not significantly so. No significant gender differences emerged for screen time.

Table 1. Health Behaviour Variables

Behaviour	*N*	Mean (SD)	Meeting guideline*(%)
Total sugary drinks (per day)	436	6.7 (4.1)	0.7
Sugar-sweetened beverages, not including milk or juice (per day)	436	3.1 (3.4)	17.9
Fruits and vegetables (per day)	433	3.2 (2.7)	10.9
Self-reported minutes of MVPA (per weekday)	428	149.7 (78.1)	91.8
Self-reported minutes of MVPA (per weekend day)	417	119.7 (102.3)	69.5
Self-reported hours of screen time (per day)	421	7.5 (4.31)	3.8
Accelerometer minutes of MVPA (per weekday)	209	58.6 (26.0)	42.1
Accelerometer minutes of MVPA (per weekend day)	260	29.0 (25.8)	11.8

*Based on recommendations from the Canada Physical Activity Guide (Canadian Society for Exercise Physiology, n.d.), Canada Food Guide for youth (Public Health Agency of Canada, 2011), and Rogers, Hart, Motyka, Rines, Vine, and Deatrick (2013), sugar-sweetened beverages: 0 servings/day, fruits and vegetables: 7-8 servings/day, MVPA: 60 minutes/day, screen time: <120 minutes/day.

Most male and female students indicated healthy eating patterns during the school week (e.g., eating breakfast); however, there was a noticeable difference in eating patterns from the weekday to the weekend. A greater percentage of youth were engaging in unhealthy eating patterns on weekends; percentages of fast food consumption, convenience snacks, and meals in front of the television were higher on weekends for both boys and girls despite eating more meals with parents on these days (Table 2). Gender differences were evident in several aspects of healthy eating: girls ate significantly more fruits and vegetables than boys, $t = -.908$, $p < 0.01$, and consumed less SSBs, $t = -6.99$, $p < .001$, while boys ate at fast food restaurants more often than girls, $t = 3.90$, $p < 0.001$, particularly on the weekend, $t = 2.79$, $p < 0.01$, and ate more convenience snacks, $t = 2.66$, $p < 0.01$.

Interpreting the results of the motivation questionnaires, we found significant correlations between both male and female students' MVPA levels and their perceived sense of skill, $r(434) = 0.17$, $p < .01$, capability, $r(434) = .015$, $p < .01$, confidence, $r(434) = 0.17$, $p < .01$, and valuing their involvement in PA, $r(434) = 0.10$, $p < .01$. Intriguingly, there was no correlation between MVPA and *understanding* how to participate in PA (Table 3).

Table 2. Eating Habits Based on the SHAPES Questionnaire

Habit	% Reporting ≥4 times during the school week (*n*)	% Reporting ≥1 time on the weekend (*n*)
Breakfast eaten	67.3 (440)	96.8 (441)
Lunch eaten	78.0 (437)	n/a
Number of times bought lunch at school	7.4 (436)	n/a
Number of times eaten at fast food restaurant	2.3 (439)	50.3 (439)
Number of times purchased vending or canteen snack	3.2 (439)	22.4 (438)
Number of times ate at school food program	2.3 (436)	n/a
Number of meals while watching TV	16.6 (440)	79.5 (440)
Number of meals eaten with an adult family member	65.1 (441)	91.6 (441)

Table 3. Correlations (*r*) between MVPA and PA Motivators Based on Values from Motivation Questionnaires

	1	2	3	4	5	6	7	8
1. MVPA minutes/ day	-	0.96**	0.84**	0.06	0.17**	0.15*	0.17**	0.10*
2. MVPA minutes/ weekday		-	0.67**	0.07	0.14**	0.13*	0.14**	0.10*
3. MVPA minutes/ weekend day			-	0.03	0.16**	0.06	0.16**	0.07
4. Understanding how to participate in PA				-	0.51**	0.62**	0.58**	0.25**
5. Feeling skilled at PA					-	0.65**	0.74**	0.21**
6. Feeling capable at PA						-	0.73**	0.28**
7. Feeling confident in PA ability							-	0.22**
8. Valuing involvement in PA								-

$*p < 0.05$, $**p < 0.01$.

Table 4. Correlations (*r*) between Sugar-sweetened Beverage (SSB) and Fruit/Vegetable (F/V) Consumption and Healthy Eating Motivators

Question	*N*	Consumption SSB (*r*)	F/V (*r*)
I don't see the point of eating healthy foods.	433	0.27**	-0.09
I don't see why I have to eat healthy.	432	0.23**	-0.15**
I try to eat healthy as little as possible.	434	0.18**	-0.126**
I eat healthy for the pleasure of eating food that is good for me.	433	-0.20**	0.270**
Eating healthy is a waste of my time.	431	0.23**	-0.04
I eat healthy because I have to.	432	0.06	-0.04
I don't see what I am getting out of eating healthy.	432	0.20**	-0.06
I eat healthy but I don't see the purpose.	433	0.14**	-0.02
I eat healthy because it is important to me.	433	-0.18**	0.18**
I have no desire to eat healthy foods.	432	0.20**	-0.14**
I eat healthy because I value my health.	433	-0.17**	0.18**
Intrinsic motivation	434	-0.19**	0.26**
Extrinsic motivation	434	0.17**	0.04

Note. Intrinsic and extrinsic motivation variables are based on summaries of healthy eating motivation questions pertaining to each motivation respectively. SSBs here do not include milk or juice. $*p < 0.05$, $**p < 0.01$.

Students reported being highly intrinsically motivated overall for eating fruits and vegetables, $r(431) = .256, p < .01$), although their motivation for consuming SSBs was found to be extrinsically driven, $r(434) = .158, p < .001$ (Table 4). We also found some subtle gender differences relating to motivation.

For intrinsic motivation, boys reported feeling more confident, $t = 6.15, p < 0.01$, and having a greater perceived skill in PE, $t = 3.16, p < 0.01$, than girls but also reported more confidence in their ability to learn in PE, $t = 1.98, p < 0.05$. Conversely, girls saw the purpose in eating healthy, $t = 2.95, p < 0.001$, viewed healthy eating as a good use of time, $t = 4.72, p < 0.001$, and viewed it as an important behaviour more than boys did, $t = 4.15, p < 0.001$.

Focus Group Results

Accessing Health Information

Students' experiences about having access to health information generated the most responses in the focus groups. Students and student Action Team members generated 236 comments related to access as it pertained to health in their lives, at their schools, and as a part of HPSS. Five subthemes within this component included a variety of topics; the number of comments related to each is stated in brackets. Not surprisingly, course material (100) was viewed as a key point of access to health education for these students across three subthemes, in particular, utilizing a variety of information sources via the classroom and having directed, health-related projects to get them thinking:

> You use like information like the library, the Internet, so you get different views again, right? Not just one singular view of like what a teacher might say, right?
>
> The HPSS assignments we did though, yeah, oh, we had to search out stuff in the community that you could do and stuff like that.

However, students felt that there were health topics that could be discussed in greater depth, primarily sexual health and mental health. As one student noted:

> Stress and coping … I think it would be better if you kind of shift gears to [having in the course] less [information on] fruit and vegetables, which we know, and maybe focus on seeing as though it is an aspect of Health 10 already. It would be a more efficient use of time.

Students on the Action Team had several suggestions pertaining to access that were related to HPSS and health in general. First, they suggested that more information (12) be provided to students via lessons and coursework: "For me personally, I think PE class shouldn't just be physical activity like running; I think that you should also like incorporate more like the kinetics of the body and like movement and how the body works."

Second, Action Team members highlighted the lack of awareness among students regarding school-wide HPSS activities and events (12) and the need to better reach students with marketing and other forms of dissemination such as social media (43): "More advertisement pages; not lots of people knew about it this year cause it's a new thing … if we were on the speaker a bit more or put signs up, more people would know more, I think."

Understanding Health Information

Student focus group participants had a great deal to say about this component of health literacy (150) while Action Team members contributed very few comments (7). A telling subtheme that emerged spoke to the redundancy or inappropriateness of health information presented in the classroom (41):

> People are saying 'manage your screen time better,' but people are literally getting their lives taken over by screen time because they are living in front of their screen. It's no longer just a matter of managing it; it's — I don't want to go so far to say — it's like a technology revolution, people! It's a thing of the past to say, 'Oh, you should manage your screen time, make sure you only have this much.' It's moving faster than the course can keep up with.
>
> There is nothing that we learned this year that we didn't already know except we did learn some new terminology, but that was it.
>
> I guess 'cause we're old enough, right, like you could sort of advance it [course material].

However, other subthemes revealed, more hopefully, students' increased understanding and growth. Specifically in both PE (79) and Health 10 (30), students changed the way they understood health behaviours. Comments related to PA changing student thinking largely related to either an increased understanding of PA (19) and its benefits or creating a broader interest in PA (33). The comments related to Health 10 as a place to become more aware of health information is evidenced by the following:

> Um, for me I have to say I really hated PE in grades eight and nine but this year I don't know if it's 'cause of our teacher or the class or the curriculum but I really like it. It's actually my favourite class this year.
>
> The teachings of PE have only made me more engaged and more interested in PA and personal health. It has wanted me to continue with PE until my senior year.
>
> [PE] has given us a lot more variety to do PA on our own; we value it more now; we have a better appreciation for it now.
>
> I think that it has extended our knowledge, and a variety of topics helped all of us in different ways. I may have thought that I was so healthy but I have learned so much … about why it is important.

Evaluating and Applying Health Information

Student focus group members were very clear in the importance and preference for aspects of health education that had real-life application (51). Students reported examples (e.g., the use of heart rate monitors, the use of weights on personal time, and CPR certification) of specific skills that could be applied outside of school to a general appreciation of knowledge relevant beyond the scope of class.

> [We] can take our new skills that we have learned and apply them to activities outside of school.
>
> I have learned techniques for different things (stretches, dance, weights, etc.) that we can use outside of school PE.

> Yeah, lots of knowledge is applicable to different fields so that's good, right, so it's not just foods and you're focusing on that but it's all different … parts of your life. So like they said careers, drugs, society, right, you should obviously learn the effects of it so that teaches you to think before you act.

While Action Team members were less concerned with evaluation and application (16), they did speak to health outcomes related to HPSS (e.g., fewer sugary drinks at the school) and increased student involvement in HPSS and health. One student Action Member noted: "The students are really enjoying this; levels of participation are increasing." Action Team members also spoke of engaging other students in creating and identifying HPSS activities for their school:

> It was good to see students initiating things and showing responsibility — it's not a class project; it is something outside which is time consuming for everyone when it's not part of your course.

Communicating Health Information

Perhaps because our focus group questions were not based on the concepts or components of health literacy, none of the focus group data were found to be overtly relevant to the communication aspect. Yet, students' engagement through their school Action Teams, and the school-wide policies and activities they implemented, suggests that they were communicating health information they saw as important for their peers and their school in a more subtle but action-oriented way. For example, Action Team members recounted several instances where health information was shared throughout their school, not through poster presentations or written class assignments, but rather by coming together in a collective decision-making process to implement:

- selling low-cost beverages on Smoothie Days in the cafeteria;
- raising monies for the Canadian Diabetes Association by having a spinning marathon with rotating classes of students participating throughout the day;
- eliminating user fees in the school weight room;
- a school-wide fruit and vegetable tasting program — once every two weeks, the school received a variety of fruit and vegetables for students to try at no cost;
- promoting Nutrition month in March; and
- partnering with local grocery stores to offer discounts on fruits and vegetables.

These activities not only required students to seek out and critically reflect on information relevant to their health but also provided interactive opportunities for students to engage in health literacy practices beyond the classroom.

DISCUSSION

Informed by the comprehensive school model, the design of HPSS was consistent with conceptual models and frameworks of health literacy that reflect and integrate multiple-levels of influencing factors at the intrapersonal, interpersonal, and community levels (Wharf Higgins, Begoray, & MacDonald, 2009). While not planned as a deliberate health literacy program, our qualitative data suggest that HPSS attended to all of the domains in the definition of health literacy: the ability to access, understand, evaluate, and communicate health information (Rootman & Gordon-El-Bihbety, 2008). Our cross-sectional look at the eating and activity practices of students as they enter secondary school confirms earlier research on gendered practices and points to the flaws remaining in the PE and health curricula. That our students were of healthy body weight is reassuring for the moment, but the intractability of lifestyle behaviours that are linked to the onset of chronic disease established at this age looms large for their future health. Recent changes to the provincial health and PE curricula (BC Ministry of Education, n.d.) that address healthy practices are to be applauded. We think that the missing link in the curricula might well be the specific inclusion of pedagogical strategies for addressing health literacy as discussed below.

We cannot dismiss students' inflated sense of their PA level, that is, self-reporting being active almost three times as much as accelerometry data revealed they actually were (Table 1). It is clearly possible that these students succumbed to social bias in over-reporting their level of PA (although this bias did not surface when conveying their sedentary and eating patterns), but it may also reflect their limited understanding of what it means to be active. In fact, correlational data from the motivation questionnaire revealed no relationship between students' activity levels and understanding how to participate in PA even though their perceived skill, confidence, and value of PA were significantly related to MVPA. Perhaps the magnified self-reported level of PA resulted from a positive attitude toward but limited understanding of what it means, literally, to be active. Indeed, students in the focus group spoke candidly about the PE curriculum enhancing their sense of value and appreciation for PA but also spoke of a desire to combine exercise (i.e., running) with learning about human movement (i.e., kinetics of the body). We contend that a health-literate person should be able to more accurately interpret their level — frequency and intensity — of PA. This may partially explain why very few youth meet the recommended levels of activity: without fully comprehending what it means to be active, they struggle to put that knowledge into action.

Unravelling these cognitive and affective components of the understanding aspect of health literacy provides an intriguing line of future research. Moreover, that boys appeared to be significantly intrinsically motivated regarding PE, and girls so for healthy eating, and that these motivational factors played out behaviourally, can inform pedagogical changes to the PE and health curricula, respectively. For example, asking students to journal their exercise and eating behaviours, including their reasons for and attitudes associated with their activity and nutrition choices, might help them to more intimately reflect on the factors influencing their health behaviours. As well, learning how to set and track behaviour change goals can engage students' cognitive function purposively rather than reacting in the moment with less healthy decisions. Linking individual decisions to the larger community, environmental, and social justice outcomes may also enhance understanding of their underlying motives for being active or eating healthfully.

Despite no gender differences in sedentary behaviours, the high level reported by our sample means that it remains an important part of the curriculum. No Action Team member selected activities or policies to address sedentary behaviour, so perhaps expanding the issue beyond the classroom is necessary to support learning in the classroom (e.g., power down days). As some of the focus group findings suggest (i.e., the students' disdain of the health education curriculum for its reprise of earlier health information), their interest and motivation to practice healthy behaviours waned. Health education in secondary school may be enhanced by engaging students in a more interactive way. While the school-wide events were intended to do just this, there may have been too few to affect any meaningful behavioural change.

Nevertheless, our findings do not belie the importance of school: interpreting the results of the motivation questionnaires provides evidence that students felt capable to be active, $r(434) = .13$, $p < .05$, and valued PA, $r(434) = .10$, $p < .05$, during the school week but not on the weekends. That consuming SSBs was extrinsically motivated supports the potency of school vending machine policies and other environmental cues that can facilitate healthy decisions in the school environment. Further, during weekends, though students reported eating more with their parents than during weekdays, they did so much less healthfully, reminding us that parents and home life play an important role in nurturing health literacy beyond the school grounds (Begoray, Wharf Higgins, & MacDonald, 2009).

In this study, as in previous research, we found that secondary school male and female students both shared and differed in their health practices. This suggests that there is a gendered nature to youth health literacy needs that should be reflected in physical and health education curricula. At the same time, a deeper understanding of the specifics of youth sedentary and screen practices can contribute to a more gender-inclusive curriculum. We are reminded of the early days of health behaviour change when *one-size-fits-all* thinking dominated interventions, holding little regard for the factors influencing personal decision making. As with the recent move toward tailoring interventions to accommodate peoples' choices, chances and circumstances, health education curricula must follow suit. Reflecting on our HPSS experience, we concur with others that the comprehensive school health approach is not comprehensive enough without addressing health literacy (Cairney et al., 2012) and, we suggest, gendered health literacy.

Because a broad mission of schools has long been to prepare students to become effective national, and more recently, global citizens (Veugelers, 2011), their learning environments need to "make a better link between what kids learn at school and what they experience and learn in their everyday lives … [and where] students can realize their full potential" (BC Ministry of Education, n.d., p. 2). Health education can tend to basic and functional health literacy; however achieving interactive health literacy demands engaging the culture and ethos of the entire school.

Questions for Discussion, Reflection, and Writing

1. In today's educational system, what do you think is the role of the school in preparing students to live healthfully? What challenges do teachers and schools face in helping their students to be healthy?
2. Do you agree with the authors that a gendered health literacy curriculum is necessary to help improve the health of male and female students? Why or why not?
3. What does this study not tell us about (gendered) adolescent health literacy?

List of Online Resources

- Begoray, D., Wharf Higgins, J., Beer, C., & Harrison, J. (2013). *Take a closer look: Media and health.* Victoria, BC: Ministry of Health. Accessed from http://www.healthyschoolsbc.ca/program/541/take-a-closer-look-media-and-health
- Centers for Disease Control and Prevention, Adolescent and School Health – http://www.cdc.gov/healthyyouth/
- Healthy Schools BC – http://www.healthyschoolsbc.ca/program/252 /dash-bc

References

American Cancer Society. (2008). *Cancer facts and figures 2008.* Atlanta, GA: Author.

Begoray, D., Wharf Higgins, J., & MacDonald, M. (2009). High school health curriculum and health literacy: Canadian student voices. *Global Health Promotion, 16*(4), 35–42.

Biddle, S. J. H., Gorely, T., Pearson, N., & Bull, F. C. (2011). An assessment of self-reported physical activity instruments in young people for population surveillance: Project ALPHA. *International Journal of Behavioral Nutrition & Physical Activity, 8*(1), 1–9.

Blanchard, C., Shilton, T., & Bull, F. (2013). Global advocacy for physical activity (GAPA): Global leadership towards a raised profile. *Global Health Promotion, 20*(4), 113–121.

Borzekowski, D. (2009). Considering children and health literacy: A theoretical approach. *Pediatrics, 124*, S282–S288.

British Columbia Ministry of Education. (n.d.). *BC's education plan.* Victoria, BC: Author. Retrieved from http://www.bcedplan.ca/assets/ pdf/bc_edu_plan.pdf

British Columbia Ministry of Health Services. (2004). *British Columbia nutrition survey: Report on food group use.* Victoria, BC: Author. Retrieved from http://www.health.gov.bc.ca/library/publications/ year/2004/bcnutritionsurvey/fgreport.pdf

British Columbia Office of the Provincial Health Officer. (2008). *An ounce of prevention revisited: A review of health promotion and selected outcomes for children and youth in BC schools. Provincial Health Officer's annual report 2006.* Victoria, BC: Ministry of Health. Retrieved from http://www.health.gov.bc.ca/pho/pdf/phoannual2006.pdf

Cairney, J., Kwan, M. Y-W., Velduizen, S., Hay, J., Bray, S. R., & Faught, B. E. (2012). Gender, perceived competence and the enjoyment of physical education in children: A longitudinal examination. *International Journal of Behavioral Nutrition and Physical Activity, 9*(26). doi:10.1186/1479-5868-9-26

Canadian Institute for Health Information. (2009). *Comparing activity and fruit and vegetable consumption by weight status among children and youth.* Ottawa, ON: Author. Retrieved from https://secure.cihi.ca/free_products/bmi_aib_e.pdf

Canadian Society for Exercise Physiology. (n.d.). *Canadian physical activity guidelines for youth - 12–17 years.* Ottawa, ON: Author. Retrieved from http://www.csep.ca/english/ view.asp?x=804

Chang, L. C. (2011). Health literacy, self-reported status and health promoting behaviours for adolescents in Taiwan. *Journal of Clinical Nursing 20*(1–2), 190–196.

Chari, R., Warsh, J., Ketterer, T., Hossain, J., & Sharif, I. (2014). Association between health literacy and child and adolescent obesity. *Patient Education and Counseling, 94*(1), 61–66.

Colley, R. C., Garriguet, D., Janssen, I., Craig, C.L., Clarke, J., & Tremblay, M. S. (2011). Physical activity of Canadian children and youth: Accelerometer results from the 2007 to 2009 Canadian Health Measures Survey. *Health Reports, 22*, 1–9.

Conwell, L. S., Callaghan, M. J., Andersen, M. J., Bor, W., Najman, J. M., & Williams, G. M. (2003). Early adolescent smoking and a web of personal and social disadvantage. *Journal of Paediatric Child Health, 39*(8), 580–585.

Coombes, E., Jones, A., Page, A., & Cooper, A. (2014). Is change in environmental supportiveness between primary and secondary school associated with a decline in children's physical activity levels? *Health & Place, 29*, 171–178.

Davis, T. C., Wolf, M. S., Arnold, C. L., Byrd, R. S., Long, S. W., Springer, T. … Bocchini, J. A. (2006). Development and validation of the Rapid Estimate of Adolescent Literacy in Medicine (REALM-Teen): A tool to screen adolescents for below-grade reading in health care settings. *Pediatrics, 188*(6), e1707–e1714.

Davis, T. C., Wolf, M. S., Bass, P. F., Middlebrooks, M., Kennen, E., Baker, D. W. … Parker, R. M. (2006). Low literacy impairs comprehension of prescription drug warning labels. *Journal of General Internal Medicine, 21*, 847–851.

Deaton, A. (2002). Policy implications of the gradient of health and wealth: An economist asks, would redistributing income improve population health? *Health Affairs, 21*, 13–30.

Deschesnes, M., Martin, C., & Jomphe Hill, A. (2003). Comprehensive approaches to school health promotion: How to achieve broader implementation? *Health Promotion International, 18*(4), 387–396.

DeWalt, D., & Hink, A. (2009). Health literacy and child health outcomes: A systematic review of the literature. *Pediatrics, 124*, S265–S274.

Esliger, D., Copeland, J., Barnes, J., & Tremblay, M. S. (2005). Standardizing and optimizing the use of accelerometer data for free living physical monitoring. *Journal of Physical Activity and Health, 3*, 366–383.

Evenson, K. R., Catellier, D. J., Gill, K., Ondrak, K. S., & McMurray, R. G. (2008). Calibration of two objective measures of physical activity for children. *Journal of Sports Sciences, 26*(14), 1557–1565.

French, S. A., Lin, B., & Guthrie, J. F. (2003). National trend in soft drink consumption among children and adolescents age 6 to 17 years: Prevalence, amounts, and sources, 1977/1978 to 1994/1998. *Journal of the American Dietetic Association, 103*(10), 1326–1331.

Gibbons, S. (2014). Relatedness-supportive learning environment for girls in physical education. *LEARNing Landscapes 7*(2), 139–150.

Gray, C. E., Barnes, J. D., Cowie Bonne, J., Cameron, C., Chaput, J-P., Faulkner, G. … Tremblay, M. S. (2014). Results from Canada's 2014 report card on PA for children and youth. *Journal of Physical Activity and Health, 11(Supp 1)*, S26–S32.

Institute of Medicine & National Research Council. (2009). *Local government actions to prevent childhood obesity*. Washington, DC: National Academies Press. Retrieved from http://www.nap.edu/catalog.php?record_id=12674

Jones, S., & Fox, S. (2009). *Generations online in 2009*. Washington, DC: Pew Research Center. Retrieved from www.pewinternet.org/~/media//Files/Reports/2009/PIP_Generations_2009.pdf

Kickbusch, I., & Maag, D. (2008). Health literacy. In K. Heggenhougen & S. Quah (Eds.), *International encyclopedia of public health* (Vol. 3, pp. 204–211). San Diego, CA: Academic Press.

Kohl, H. W., Craig, C. L., Lambert, E. V., Inoue, S., Ramadan Alkandari, J., Leetongin, G., & Khalmeier, S. (2012). The pandemic of physical inactivity: Global action for public health. *The Lancet, 380*(9838), 294–305.

Kriemler, S., Meyer, U., Martin, E., van Sluijs, E. M. F., Andersen, B., & Martin, B. W. (2011). Effect of school-based interventions on physical activity and fitness in children and adolescents: A review of reviews and systematic update. *British Journal of Sports Medicine, 45*, 923–930.

Levin-Zamir, D., Lemish, D., & Gofin, R. (2011). Media health literacy (MHL): Development and measurement of the concept among adolescents. *Health Education Research, 26*(2), 323–335.

Manganello, J. (2008). Health literacy and adolescents: A framework and agenda for future research. *Health Education Research, 23*(5), 840–847.

Markland, D., & Tobin, V. (2004). A modification to the behavioral regulation in exercise questionnaire to include an assessment of amotivation. *Journal of Sport & Exercise Psychology, 26*, 191–196.

Marks, R., & Wharf Higgins, J. (2012). Healthy literacy skills needed by children, teachers and parents. In R. Marks (Ed.), *Health literacy and school-based health education* (pp. 63–77). Bingley, England: Emerald.

Massey, P., Prelip, M., Calimlim, B., Afifi, A., Quiter, E., Nessim, S. … Glik, D. (2013). Findings toward a multidimensional measure of adolescent health literacy. *American Journal of Health Behavior, 37*(3), 342–350.

Molt, R. W., McAuley, E., Birnbaum, A. S., & Lytle, L. A. (2006). Naturally occurring changes in time spent watching television are inversely related to frequency of physical activity during early adolescence. *Journal of Adolescence, 29*(1), 19–32.

Naylor, P. J., Macdonald, H. M., Warburton, D. E. R., Reed, K. E., & McKay, H. A. (2008). An active school model to promote physical activity in elementary schools: Action schools! BC. *British Journal of Sports Medicine, 42*(5), 338–343.

Norman, C. D., & Skinner, H. A. (2006). eHeals: The eHealth literacy scale. *Journal of Medical Internet Research, 8*(4), e27.

Orji, R., Vassileva, J., & Mandryk, R. (2013). Modeling gender differences in healthy eating determinants for persuasive intervention design. In S. Berkovsky & J. Frenye (Eds.), *Persuasive technology, lecture notes in computer science* (pp. 161–173). Berlin, Germany: Springer-Verlag.

Ormshaw, M. J., Paakkari, L., & Kannas, L. K. (2013). Measuring child and adolescent health literacy: A systematic review of literature. *Health Education, 113*(5), 433–455.

Paakkari, L., & Paakkari, O. (2012). Health literacy as a learning outcome in schools. *Health Education, 112*(2), 133–152.

Patton, M. Q. (2002). *Qualitative research and evaluation methods* (3rd ed.). Thousand Oaks, CA: SAGE.

Pearson, N., & Biddle, S. (2011). Sedentary behavior and dietary intake in children, adolescents, and adults. A systematic review. *American Journal of Preventive Medicine, 41*(2), 178–188.

Perry, E. L. (2014). Health literacy in adolescents: An integrative review. *Journal for Specialists in Pediatric Nursing, 19*(3), 210–218.

Public Health Agency of Canada. (2011). *Eating well with Canada's food guide*. Ottawa, ON: Health Canada. Retrieved from: http://www.hc-sc.gc.ca/fn-an/alt_formats/hpfb-dgpsa/pdf/food-guide-aliment/view_eatwell_vue_bienmang-eng.pdf

Pujazon-Zazik, M., & Park, M. J. (2010). To tweet, or not to tweet: Gender differences and potential positive and negative health outcomes of adolescents' social internet use. *American Journal of Men's Health, 4*(1), 77–85.

Raine, K. D. (2004). *Overweight and obesity in Canada: A population health perspective.* Ottawa, ON: Canadian Institute for Health Information. Retrieved from https://secure.cihi.ca/free_products/CPHIOverweightandObesityAugust2004_e.pdf

Robertson, W., Stewart-Brown, S., Wilcock, E., Oldfield, M., & Thorogood, M. (2011). Utility of accelerometers to measure physical activity in children attending an obesity treatment intervention. *Journal of Obesity, 2011*, Article 398918.

Rogers, V., Hart, P., Motyka, E., Rines, E., Vine, J., & Deatrick, D. (2013). Impact of let's go! 5-2-1-0: A community-based, multisetting childhood obesity prevention program. *Journal of Pediatric Psychology, 38*(9), 1010–1020.

Rootman, I., & Gordon-El-Bihbety, D. (2008). *A vision for a health literate Canada: Report of the expert panel on health literacy*. Ottawa, ON: Canadian Public Health Association. Retrieved from http://www.cpha.ca/uploads/portals/h-l/report_e.pdf

Rovner, A., Nansel, T., Wang, J., & Iannotti, R. (2011). Foods sold in school vending machines are associated with overall student dietary intake. *Journal of Adolescent Health, 48*(1), 13–19.

Simonds, S. K. (1974). Health education as social policy. *Health Education Monographs, 2*(1), 1.

Sorenson, K., Van den Broucke, S., Fullam, J., Doyle, G., Pelikan, J., Slonska, Z. … HLS-EU Consortium. (2012). Health literacy and public health: A systematic review and integration of definitions and models. *BMC Public Health, 12*(80). doi:10.1186/1471-2458-12-80

St. Leger, L. (2001). Schools, health literacy and public health: Possibilities, overlaps and challenges. *Health Promotion International, 16*(2), 197–205.

Stone, E. J., McKenzie, T. L., Welk, G. J., & Booth, M. L. (1998). Effects of physical activity interventions in youth: Review and synthesis. *American Journal of Preventative Medicine, 15*(4), 298–315.

Story, M., Kaphingst, K. M., & French, S. (2006). The role of schools in obesity prevention. *Future Child, 16*(1), 109–142.

Tremblay, M. S., Shields, M., Laviolette, M., Craig, C. L., Janssen, I., & Connor Gorber, S. (2010). Fitness of Canadian children and youth: Results from the 2007-2009 Canadian Health Measures Survey (Statistics Canada 82-003-X). *Health Reports, 21*(1). Retrieved from http://www.statcan.gc.ca/pub/82-003-x/2010001/article/11065-eng.htm

Veugelers, W. (2011). The moral and the political in global citizenship: Appreciating differences in education. *Globalisation, Societies and Education, 9*(3-4), 473–485.

Wharf Higgins, J., Begoray, D., & MacDonald, M. (2009). A social ecological conceptual framework for understanding adolescent health literacy in the health education classroom. *American Journal of Community Psychology, 44*(3–4), 350–362.

Wharf Higgins, J., Bellows Riecken, K., Voss, C., Naylor, P. J., Gibbons, S., Rhodes, R. … McKay, H. (2013). Health promoting secondary schools: Community-based research examining voice, choice, and the school setting. *Journal of Child and Adolescent Behavior*, *1*(3). doi:10.4172/jcalb.1000118

Wharf Higgins, J., Gaul, C., Gibbons, S., & Van Gyn, G. (2003). Factors influencing physical activity levels among Canadian youth. *Canadian Journal of Public Health, 94*(1), 45–51.

Wharf Higgins, J., Naylor, P. J., Bellows Riecken, K., Gibbons, S., Rhodes, R., Sulz, L., & McKay, H. (2014). One, two, three strikes and you're out? Examining youth physical activity in the context of the health promoting secondary schools model and teacher job action. *Education and Health, 32*(3), 110–117.

Wu, A. D., Begoray, D., MacDonald, M., Wharf Higgins, J., Frankish, J., Kwan, B. … Rootman, I. (2010). Measuring health literacy of Canadian high school students. *Health Promotion International*, *25*(4), 444–452.

In: Adolescent Health Literacy and Learning
Editors: D. L. Begoray and E. M. Banister
ISBN: 978-1-63482-897-0

Chapter 7

INTEGRATING CULTURE TO ENHANCE MENTAL HEALTH LITERACY AMONG ABORIGINAL YOUTH

E. Anne Marshall*
Department of Educational Psychology and Leadership Studies,
University of Victoria, Canada

ABSTRACT

Aboriginal youth report much higher rates of mental health and substance abuse problems than non-Aboriginal youth, yet they often do not seek help or treatment. A frequently cited reason for this situation is that these youth lack *mental health literacy* – they may not have sufficient knowledge to identify mental health symptoms and/or they may not know how to access mental health support and treatment. Additional barriers to help-seeking include discrimination and stigma, problems with treatment access, lack of cultural safety, and the intergenerational negative impacts of colonization. In order to improve mental health outcomes for Aboriginal youth, culturally and contextually appropriate strategies and resources to increase mental health literacy are needed for both the youth themselves and for those educators, professionals, and other adult allies working with them. Culturally relevant and culturally safe mental health approaches, programs, and resources can engage and empower Aboriginal youth to recognize their strengths and support them along the path of mental wellness.

Keywords: Aboriginal youth, Aboriginal youth mental health literacy, Aboriginal culture, mental health education, mental health literacy, stigma, youth mental health

* Corresponding author: Email: amarshal@uvic.ca.

INTRODUCTION

Focusing Questions

1. How is mental health literacy different for Aboriginal youth than for non-Aboriginal youth?
2. Why is it important that adults who work with Aboriginal youth have some knowledge and understanding about Aboriginal culture and the history of colonization?

Mental health problems affect about one in five youth and young adults today, according to several research estimates (Bourget & Chenier, 2007; Jorm, Morgan, & Wright, 2008; Mood Disorders Society of Canada, 2009; Wile Schwartz, 2009). Effective treatments are available; however, research indicates that less than half of those with a mental health problem access mental health services (Marcus & Westra, 2012; Pinto-Foltz, Logsdon, & Myers, 2011). Of those who seek treatment, factors such as lack of information, accessibility, and mental illness stigma have been linked to premature termination (Pinto-Foltz et al., 2011). Thus, as a group, young people have a high rate of unmet mental health care needs. The situation, however, is even more problematic for Aboriginal youth. In this chapter, *Aboriginal* is meant to include all original or indigenous peoples. In Canada, they may identify as First Nations, Metis, Inuit, or Non-Status Indian; in the United States, many identify as Native American. In this chapter, authors' terms have been retained as used in the literature.

Although Aboriginal youth represent less than 20% of the youth and young adult population in Canada and the United States, they report much higher rates of mental health and substance abuse problems than non-Aboriginal youth (Price & Dalgleish, 2013; Public Health Agency of Canada, 2006). Health care and education professionals have been advocating for an increased focus on mental health prevention and interventions that are specifically tailored for Aboriginal and other adolescents (Potvin-Boucher & Malone, 2014; Thira, 2014). Moreover, mental health practitioners and researchers have recommended that teachers, counselors, and other adults who work with youth acquire the knowledge and skills to support them to seek help for mental and emotional difficulties (Pinfold, Stuart, Thornicroft, & Arboleda-Flórez, 2005; Whitley, Smith, & Vaillancourt, 2013).

A frequently cited reason for youth not seeking help for mental health problems is that they lack *mental health literacy* — they may not have sufficient knowledge to identify mental health symptoms and/or they may not know how to access mental health support and treatment (Jorm et al., 2008; Marcus & Westra, 2012). For Aboriginal youth, Kirmayer, Simpson, and Cargo (2003) and Smye, Browne, and Josewski (2010) have observed that additional barriers to help-seeking (e.g., discrimination and stigma, problems with treatment access, and lack of cultural safety) often exist. In order to improve mental health outcomes for Aboriginal youth, these authors maintain that culturally and contextually appropriate strategies and resources to increase mental health literacy (MHL) are needed for both the youth themselves and for those working with them.

Improving MHL among Aboriginal adolescents, as well as among the adults who support them, is critically important for several reasons. First, Aboriginal populations tend to be relatively young; there are proportionately more Aboriginal young people than non-

Aboriginal in many countries. In Canada, for example, Aboriginal youth aged 15 to 24 years comprise about 18% of the total Aboriginal population nationally as compared to about 13% for non-Aboriginal youth (Statistics Canada, 2013a). The figures are similar in the United States (United States Census Bureau, 2012), and demographers agree that Aboriginal populations worldwide are increasing at greater rates than non-Aboriginal (Statistics Canada, 2013b).

Second, the reported incidence of mental health problems among Aboriginal people in general — and among Aboriginal youth in particular — is higher than for non-Aboriginal youth (Health Canada, 2011; Price & Dalgleish, 2013; Westerman, 2010). Depression rates for Aboriginal people who live off reserve, for example, are one and one-half times higher than for the non-Aboriginal population in Canada (Mood Disorders Society, 2009). Anxiety, mood disorders, and substance abuse are also reported more frequently for Aboriginal people (Potvin-Boucher & Malone, 2014). The figures for suicide are particularly alarming; Aboriginal youth suicide rates are up to five times higher than rates for non-Aboriginal youth (Chandler & Lalonde, 2008; Kirmayer et al., 2003; Price & Dalgleish, 2013).

The third reason for heightened concern for Aboriginal youth mental health is that at least half of those who develop a mental health problem experience their first episode before the age of 18 years (Chalmers et al., 2014). Because risks can be heightened at this developmentally sensitive time, early intervention can provide long-term benefits by preventing the worsening of mental health problems later (Reavley & Jorm, 2011a). The dual intent of mental health literacy — education and prevention — is consistent with adolescent developmental pathways. Because of historical and colonization factors, however, Aboriginal youth have particular cultural needs that must be considered for mental health education and interventions (Lopes, Lindeman, Taylor, & Grant, 2012; Nagel, Thompson, Robinson, Condon, & Trauer, 2009; Potvin-Boucer & Malone, 2014).

In this chapter, a cultural approach is suggested as an important ingredient in any program or strategy addressing Aboriginal youth mental health literacy. First, a snapshot of youth mental health figures is presented, with particular emphasis on Aboriginal youth. Next is a discussion of MHL, youth MHL in general, and MHL related to Aboriginal youth that highlights three key aspects. Education and training considerations are presented, including the popular mental health first aid (MHFA) approach. Several resources and programs aimed at increasing youth MHL are briefly described as examples that have been successfully implemented. The chapter concludes with suggestions and implications for practice and research.

Youth Mental Health

Approximately one in five adolescents and young adults in North America between the ages of 15 and 24 years have reported a mental health and/or substance abuse problem (Marcus & Westra, 2012; Mood Disorders Society, 2009; Wile Schwartz, 2009). Figures are similar for young people in Australia, New Zealand, and the United Kingdom (Jorm et al., 2008; youthbeyondblue, 2015). Depression and anxiety are the most common problems, with young women often reporting higher rates than young men. Conduct disorders, attention deficit-hyperactivity disorders, psychoses, and substance use disorders are less frequent but on the increase according to some studies (Chalmers et al., 2014).

Even though the incidence of mental health problems among the general youth population is of concern, more alarming are the findings for Aboriginal youth. Researchers in Canada have found that 75% of Aboriginal community residents report youth alcohol and substance use as a problem within their community, with figures as high as 48% cannabis use in the 15–17-year-old category (Public Health Agency, 2006). In their survey of Aboriginal youth mental health, the First Nations Health Council (2003) found that 21% of youth reported feeling sad, blue, or depressed for more than two weeks in a row, 20% reported contemplating suicide, 18% experienced the suicide of a close relation, and almost 50% reported regular use of alcohol. Aboriginal youth suicide rates are acknowledged to be the highest in the world (Chandler & Lalonde, 2008); North American estimates range from 22% to 38% (Center for Native American Youth, n.d.; Health Canada, 2011). Suicide and self-inflicted injuries are the leading cause of death among Aboriginal young people in Canada (Public Health Agency, 2006) and Australia (youthbeyondblue, 2015), and the third leading cause in the United States (Wile Schwartz, 2009). These figures underscore the need for treatment and prevention programs and strategies to address mental health and mental illness among Aboriginal youth. A focus on improving mental health literacy for both youth and adults who work with youth represents an important step to achieving this.

Mental Health Literacy

Definitions

Mental health literacy, a relatively recent concept, is a more specific aspect of the broader notion of health literacy in general. The first widely accepted definition of MHL — "mental health literacy comprises the knowledge, beliefs and abilities that enable the recognition, management or prevention of mental health problems" — was proposed by the Australian psychiatrist Anthony Jorm and his colleagues (Jorm, 1997, p. 183). Just as inadequate health literacy results in negative health outcomes and increases the burden and costs associated with disease, a lack of mental health literacy is similarly suggested to negatively affect understanding, recognition, and treatment-seeking for mental illnesses. Moreover, the stigma associated with mental illness has been identified as a major barrier to help-seeking, both for those who suffer as well as for family and friends (Marcus & Westra, 2012). Jorm and his colleagues (Jorm, 2000; Jorm et al., 1997; Jorm et al., 2008) argued that improving MHL among professionals and the general public should be a key strategy for improving mental health overall. They and other researchers have conducted several investigations to identify barriers, supports, and factors that affect MHL; several youth-related examples are described later in this chapter.

Since its introduction, numerous studies and evaluations have used Jorm's definition, focusing largely on the identification, description, and interventions related to specific mental health disorders such as depression and psychosis (Jorm, Christensen, & Griffiths, 2005; Marcus & Westra, 2012). National surveys in Australia investigated how well people could identify disorders from short descriptive vignettes (Jorm et al., 2005). Initially, researchers generally found that many people had poor MHL; that is, they did not recognize common mental health problems, they did not know about treatments or their effectiveness, they had negative attitudes about seeking help for mental health problems, and they could not assist others to recognize problems or get appropriate help (Jorm et al., 1997). This led to public awareness, information, and education campaigns, such as *beyondblue* (2015), that have resulted in overall improvements in MHL over the past several years (Jorm et al., 2005).

In a report to the Canadian Alliance on Mental Illness and Mental Health (CAMIMH) Bourget and Chenier (2007) proposed a broader definition of MHL: "mental health literacy is the knowledge and skills that enable people to access, understand and apply information for mental health" (p. 4). This definition puts more emphasis on empowerment, an important concept in health promotion and health literacy. Using this definition, enhancing MHL involves more than providing people with information about symptoms and treatment options; it includes support for skill development and empowerment in order that people are able not only to understand information but also to make informed decisions and take effective action to promote positive mental health for themselves and others (Bourget & Chenier, 2007). Those with high levels of MHL are better able to identify mental health "strengths and needs in themselves and others, are better equipped and more empowered to seek appropriate supports, and report lower levels of mental health stigma" (Potvin-Boucher & Malone, 2014, p. 346). This approach to MHL includes an emphasis on the key role of professionals and practitioners who are in contact with people experiencing mental health difficulties and, therefore, in a position to offer information and support.

Youth MHL

Increasing MHL has become a goal in many countries over the past two decades with evidence of success (e.g., Jorm et al., 2005). Few studies, however, have explored MHL related to youth populations; even fewer have included Aboriginal youth. This raises concern as existing research suggests low rates of MHL in youth and young adults (Pinto-Foltz et al., 2011). A few studies with youth are summarized below.

In Australia, Reavley and Jorm (2011a, 2011b) conducted a computer-assisted national telephone survey focusing on mental health literacy and stigma with 3,021 young people aged 15–25 years (no cultural identity information was provided). Respondents were read one of six case vignettes portraying a young person (named John or Jenny) with depression, depression with suicidal thoughts, psychosis, social phobia, depressions with alcohol abuse, or post traumatic stress disorder (PTSD); they were then asked a series of questions about mental health literacy (e.g., "What do you think is wrong with John/Jenny?"), stigma, exposure to mental disorders, and beliefs about interventions. Of the respondents, 75% recognized depression while about one-third recognized psychosis (e.g., schizophrenia) and PTSD. Family members were named as the most likely source of help across all six vignettes. Reavley and Jorm concluded that most young people's MHL for recognizing signs of depression was good; however, it was much lower for other disorders; and there was a tendency to overgeneralize the term *depression*. In addition, there was considerable reluctance to endorse professional help-seeking for mental health problems, indicating that stigma continues to be a limiting factor. The authors recommended more emphasis on MHL education and media information in order to promote increased mental health knowledge among youth and a reduction of the stigma associated with mental health problems.

In a Canadian study, Marcus and Westra (2012) analyzed the responses of 123 young adults aged 18–24 years who were part of a 2006 computer-assisted MHL telephone survey (*N* = 1,004) conducted by the CAMIMH. The survey began with a short vignette of a person (named Robert or Mary) suffering from depression, anxiety, or schizophrenia (psychosis). Participants were then asked questions about problem recognition, knowledge about mental illness, possible causes, and management or treatment options. Marcus and Westra found no significant difference between younger and older adults in terms of rates of recognition and mental health knowledge, with higher rates of depression recognition (~80%) in contrast to anxiety or schizophrenia (~50%); there were few differences related to causal beliefs between the age groups. However, with respect to treatment, young adults were significantly less in favour of accessing professional care (e.g., family doctor), less likely to view medications as helpful, and marginally less likely to believe that psychotherapy could be helpful. These young adults, especially young men, reported more interest in managing mental health problems either on their own or with the support of friends or family. The authors recommended development of MHL interventions aimed at help-seeking behaviours, attitudes about treatment options, and "alternative youth-friendly options for managing mental health problems" (Marcus & Westra, 2012, p. 10).

In a U.S study, McCarthy, Bruno, and Fernandes (2011) investigated adolescent MHL with a group of high school students (*N* = 36) using vignettes depicting depression and suicidality. They found that the teens were able to differentiate depressed from nondepressed vignettes and could identify (a) common symptoms of depression and (b) sources of help that varied according to the perceived degree of problem severity. The authors recommended including adolescents more actively when planning and providing mental health education or treatment services. They suggested that additional research is needed with culturally diverse groups since understanding of mental health risks, behaviours, and help-seeking is affected by cultural values, beliefs, and practices. As discussed in the next section, cultural factors are particularly salient for Aboriginal youth.

Aboriginal Youth MHL

A number of scholars and researchers assert that understanding and addressing mental health needs and MHL among Aboriginal populations require a cultural approach that recognizes the historical and continuing impacts of colonization and assimilation policies that have had and continue to have profound negative effects on the physical, emotional, mental, and spiritual wellbeing of Indigenous peoples worldwide (Kirmayer et al., 2003; Nuttgens & Campbell, 2010; Potvin-Boucher & Malone, 2014; Thira, 2014). Rather than constituting a health crisis within an individual, mental health problems are seen as a *community crisis* with social, political, and economic causes that call for a cultural *cure* that is "rooted in the reclaiming of wellness through the contemporary expression of traditional values" (Thira, 2014, p. 158). A post-colonial approach is recommended — one that recognizes the importance of Indigenous worldviews and values, ancestral and kinship connections, the role of community, a holistic understanding of wellness that includes spirituality, and the intergenerational impacts of colonization (Marshall et al., 2014; Nuttgens & Campbell, 2010).

To foster enhanced MHL for Aboriginal youth, Potvin-Boucher & Malone (2014) suggested three elements to be considered: address historical and cultural factors, promote youth engagement, and facilitate youth empowerment. Each of these will be discussed briefly.

Aboriginal cultures are diverse; however, there are a number of shared beliefs that warrant recognition in order to understand the Aboriginal context: the importance of spirituality, the interconnectedness of life, the role of elders and knowledge keepers, the use of stories to teach life lessons, and connection to the land (Kanowski, Jorm, & Hart, 2009; Potvin-Boucher & Malone, 2014; Thira, 2014). Teachers, professionals, and other adults who interact with Aboriginal youth need to understand the history of colonization and assimilation practices that have negatively affected Indigenous families and communities for generations. Residential schooling, adoption of Aboriginal children, forced migration from traditional lands, outlawing of potlatch ceremonies, and loss of Aboriginal status have had devastating effects on individuals and families (Kirmayer et al., 2003; Nuttgens & Campbell, 2010). The effects of these widespread policies have been linked to the higher incidence of substance misuse and mental health problems experienced in Aboriginal communities together with a mistrust of colonial or western treatment methods (Lopes et al., 2012). Thira (2014) recounted that an Aboriginal colleague once asked him, "How can you [the colonizer] offer the cure when you are the disease?" (p. 161). Although the negative impacts are clear, it is important to note that strength, resilience, community mobilization, and stories of resistance exist – these positive factors can inspire Aboriginal youth to reclaim and connect with their culture in ways that promote positive mental health (Chandler & Lalonde, 2008; Price & Dalgleish, 2013). In terms of youth mental health treatment and healing, an integration of traditional and western methods or two-way approaches can be successful, particularly since youth *walk in two worlds* and many live in off-reserve urban environments (Nagel et al., 2009; Potvin-Boucher & Malone, 2014). As part of addressing historical and cultural factors, educators and professionals should incorporate local history, knowledge, language, and customs that will be familiar to Aboriginal youth and communities.

Promoting Aboriginal youth engagement in MHL, the second element, includes fostering an understanding of cultural past and present that acknowledges strengths and overcoming obstacles; this can be a precursor to developing a sense of cultural identity and pride (Potvin-Boucher & Malone, 2014). Traditional teachings and ways of knowing within Aboriginal cultures emphasize hands-on approaches, land-based activities, community rituals, and ceremonies. Teachers, counselors, and mental health professionals can work with elders and knowledge keepers to help youth learn skills such as traditional food gathering and preparation in concert with language and ceremonies (Marshall et al., 2014). Mentoring and leadership activities can build teamwork and healthy relationships that foster a sense of belonging and self-esteem — key aspects of positive mental health. Opportunities to engage in art, singing, and storytelling activities help develop skills while facilitating youth's learning of culture and language (Lopes et al., 2012).

Facilitating youth empowerment to make healthy choices is the third element to consider in MHL. Potvin-Boucher and Malone (2014) suggest that respect is a key aspect to incorporate as well as the belief that everyone takes responsibility for their actions; empowering Aboriginal youth "to make healthy decisions has the potential to reduce high-risk behaviours and increase mental wellness" (p. 350). Choosing to ask for help from peers and adult allies and viewing this as a sign of strength can address the problem of stigma or shame associated with needing and seeking help for mental health difficulties (Nagel et al., 2009).

The above discussion has underscored the importance of culture, engagement, and empowerment as the elements needed to promote and improve MHL among Aboriginal youth. The next section focuses on how to foster MHL among the teachers, counselors, and other professionals who support these youth.

Enhancing Professionals' Mental Health Literacy

There are a number of principles and practices that have been demonstrated to be effective for teachers, counselors, mental health practitioners, and other adult allies who wish to enhance their own MHL knowledge and skills to work more effectively with Aboriginal youth (Whitley et al., 2013). These include establishing cultural safety, implementing mental health first aid practices, and addressing stigma. Each of these will be discussed briefly.

Cultural Safety

Cultural safety is essential to any discussion of Aboriginal MHL; culturally safe practices recognize and respect the cultural identities of others and safely meet needs, expectations, and rights (Brascoupé & Waters, 2009). People understand mental health in culturally bound ways, yet this is not always acknowledged in mainstream mental health education and service delivery (Chalmers et al., 2014; Health Canada, 2011; Pinto-Foltz et al., 2011). Numerous researchers have identified more help-seeking barriers for Aboriginal than for non-Aboriginal people (Health Canada, 2011; Reavley & Jorm, 2011b; Smye et al., 2010), including a history of racism and discrimination, a resulting lack of trust in mainstream services, misunderstandings due to cultural and language differences, and a lack of adequate measures to reduce the stigma associated with mental illnesses (Chalmers et al., 2014). A lack of cultural safety is one explanation for this reluctance to seek help.

Cultural safety includes both process and outcome (Ramsden, 1990). As a *process*, cultural safety provides a critical lens to address the unequal power relations that have shaped much of education and health services delivered to Aboriginal and other minority populations. Professionals need to become aware of how power and privilege operates in their relationships and to understand Aboriginal views of mental health, family, and community. Signs and symptoms of mental illness should be discussed within a cultural context, and specialized cultural adaptations of health education programs are appropriate. Achieving the *outcome* of cultural safety involves adopting culturally sensitive and respectful attitudes, education, and practices and making cultural adaptations to health education programs (Brascoupé & Waters, 2009; Smye et al., 2010). Cultural safety principles have been incorporated into training and educational curricula for both professional and lay helpers and need to be a component of any mental health program with Aboriginal youth (Lopes et al., 2009).

Mental Health First Aid (MHFA) Practices

MHFA is an increasingly popular approach to improving mental health literacy; it is based on the familiar practice of providing first aid in physical health situations and is defined as "the help provided to a person who appears to be developing a mental health problem or in a mental health crisis" (Kitchener & Jorm, 2008, p. 55). MHFA training includes the following: attitudes, knowledge, and beliefs that help in recognizing, managing, and preventing mental illnesses; how to recognize specific disorders; knowing how to find mental health information; understanding risk factors and causes; how to promote appropriate help-seeking; and learning about self-help strategies and what professional help is available. Originally intended for a broad range of public audiences, specialized versions have subsequently been developed for educators, helping professionals, first responders, youth workers, and cultural groups, including Aboriginal adults and youth (Kanowski et al., 2009). MHFA has been adapted and implemented in 15 countries (Health Canada, 2011). Evaluation studies have consistently demonstrated that completion of a MHFA training experience results in positive changes in MHL, knowledge and use of first aid skills, and decreases in mental health stigma (Ganshorn & Michaud, 2012; Kitchener & Jorm, 2008).

The action-oriented *first aid* aspect of MHFA is captured in the acronym ALGEE: **A**ssess risk of suicide or harm, **L**isten nonjudgmentally, **G**ive reassurance and information, **E**ncourage the person to get appropriate professional help, and **E**ncourage self-help strategies. These five principles can be applied to a variety of mental health problems, including depression and anxiety. The principles are also appropriate for less serious situations and have been adapted for use in schools and community settings (Caza, 2010; Health Canada, 2011).

Youth mental health first aid (YMHFA) is a variation of the standard MHFA course that is specifically designed to improve the mental health literacy of adult service providers who work with adolescents (Kelly et al., 2011). The YMHFA program emphasizes the importance of early intervention in order to minimize the impact of mental health problems on adolescent development. An evaluation of the program indicated improvements in participants' knowledge, attitudes, and helping behaviours (Kelly et al., 2011). A further adaptation of the training program was designed specifically for assisting Aboriginal and Torres Strait Islander Australians (Kanowski et al., 2009). Historical, cultural, and political forces affecting Aboriginal mental health were recognized in the course; Aboriginal people understand mental health within a cultural framework that does not always fit with western methods.

In a recent study by Chalmers et al. (2014), a panel of youth mental health professionals was able to reach consensus about culturally appropriate communication strategies for providing YMHFA for Aboriginal adolescents. They recommended several guidelines, including incorporating cultural influences, using appropriate communication, discussing options with youth, and handling difficulties. A number of barriers to accessing service that need to be addressed were identified, such as language, mobility, discrimination, and shame. Empowering Aboriginal adolescents to make informed choices about seeking mental health assistance was a strong theme in the program across this diverse group of practitioners.

Addressing Stigma

Myths about mental illness comprise a significant part of mental health illiteracy (Health Canada, 2011; Jorm et al., 2008). These myths lead to stigmatizing beliefs and attitudes that result in discrimination toward people with mental health difficulties. Stigma related to mental illness has been studied for almost 50 years yet continues to be a major hurdle in the help-seeking process. Therefore, challenging the underlying myths of stigma is a significant component of promoting positive MHL. Professionals need to understand the multiple aspects of stigma and to develop strategies to combat cultural and other stereotypes that undermine positive mental health attitudes (Health Canada, 2011).

Resources to Support Aboriginal Youth MHL

There is a growing number of interventions and programs that aim to reduce mental illness stigma and improve MHL among children and adolescents (Pinto-Foltz et al., 2011), including school-based curricula, knowledge-contact initiatives, multimedia tools, online resources, and theatrical drama. Several examples are described below; all have cultural components, and a few have been developed specifically for Aboriginal youth.

The Healthy Aboriginal Network (2014) is a nonprofit society established in British Columbia in 2005 with the goal of promoting of health, literacy, and wellness for Aboriginal young people through the production of visual resources: graphic novels (similar to comic books), DVDs, posters, and augmented reality knowledge transfer — a process that uses a special mobile phone application to trigger videos and additional information. One graphic novel entitled "Just a Story" is about mental health stigma; another entitled "Lost Innocence" is about the impacts of residential schools. These graphic novels can be used with individual youth in counselling and health service contexts as well as with groups in schools, cultural programs, and community organizations.

Another program, a national initiative to address issues associated with depression, anxiety and related disorders called *beyondblue* (2015), was established in Australia in 2000. The beyondblue four-part message is understand, do something, help someone, and get involved. The main website provides general information; there is a separate page for all young people aged 16–24 years called *youthbeyondblue* and a separate section for Aboriginal and Torres Strait Islander peoples that includes youth. The user-friendly website offers a 24-hour helpline, online chats, information, apps, downloadable resources, videos, and links to people's stories.

The Pan-Canadian Joint Consortium for School Health (Morrison & Peterson, 2015) has created a "Positive Mental Health Toolkit" to promote positive mental health perspectives and practices for youth in school contexts (see http://www.jcshpositivementalhealthtoolkit.com). The Toolkit is based on evidence-informed practice and intended to facilitate a process for engaging school and community strengths to support youth mental wellbeing in the broader sense. The Toolkit is paired with a "Better Practices" document that includes information, activities, and resources for all school levels.

An intervention entitled "In Our Own Voice" (National Alliance on Mental Illness [NAMI], n.d.) is designed to improve MHL and reduce stigma (Pinto-Foltz et al., 2011). Administered by NAMI in the United States, this program uses narrative storytelling, discussion, and a video presentation and lasts about one hour (see www.nami.org). Initial evaluations of the intervention have demonstrated some efficacy with regard to improving MHL and reducing stigma among adolescents and young adults.

"Through the Pain to Wellness" is a week-long workshop that was initially developed to address the problem of Aboriginal youth suicide (Thira, 2014). Over the past 15 years, it has been expanded for a broader range of mental health problems and adapted for non-Aboriginal and mixed communities. It follows a three-step model of post-colonial consciousness raising, youth crisis intervention, and cultural values-based community development. The purpose of the workshop is to engage community capacity to improve individual, family, and community wellness. Elder participation and traditional knowledge are key components of the program.

Fostering a Climate for Learning

Developing a positive, engaging climate for learning is important when considering sensitive and emotion-focused topics such as Aboriginal MHL (Westerman, 2010; Whitley et al., 2013). In addition to culturally appropriate content, educators need to draw on their extensive knowledge and skills related to youth ways of communicating and learning. Peer relationships are paramount with adolescents, yet they also look to teachers as knowledgeable adults they can trust. Youth-friendly communication styles and avoiding assumptions can facilitate the discussion of mental health topics. Since youth today spend much of their time online, digital formats are a good way to engage their attention. A few suggestions are highlighted below.

As Moses (2010) observed, mental health information and treatment-seeking among adolescents is significantly influenced by the opinions of peers and influential adults in their social network. Adolescents often prefer to discuss mental health issues with their peers but may be reluctant to do so because they anticipate negative responses and stigmatization (Jorm et al., 2008; Pinto-Foltz et al., 2011). Because mental health beliefs and mental health stigma are grounded in social relationships and contexts, it is important to establish a climate of openness and acceptance in the classroom and other learning environments. In recent research with mental health practitioners who worked with Aboriginal youth (Marshall et al., 2014), acceptance, relationship building, and trust were universally endorsed as essential for success.

Professionals need to adopt youth-friendly communication approaches when attempting to engage Aboriginal youth. Westerman (2010) outlined an 11-step model of engagement for Aboriginal youth in mental health treatment that has been tested with rural and urban youth. It includes elements such as relationship building, choosing appropriate locations for conversation, sitting side by side with youth, acknowledging nonverbal expressions, being aware of belief systems, and having access to a cultural consultant. Westerman acknowledged that particular or local contexts have specific values, expectations, and practices; however, she maintained that the model has universal elements that can be adapted or extended by mental health service providers to fit the diversity of Aboriginal cultures. Although developed for mental health practitioners, teachers can easily implement most of the steps.

Though each person's context is to some extent unique, Aboriginal young people have much in common with their non-Aboriginal counterparts because of developmental and contextual similarities. Non-Aboriginal teachers and other allies can sometimes feel uncomfortable when discussing topics such as colonization and discrimination (Nuttgens &

Campbell, 2010). However, Chalmers et al. (2014) found that helping professionals endorsed many of the same communication practices with Aboriginal adolescents that were used with non-Aboriginal adolescents; for example, asking where they feel comfortable and safe to talk, taking time to build rapport and trust, being reliable and consistent, listening without interrupting, being genuine, talking calmly, having awareness of body language, and offering courses of action. Many educators and helpers who have experience with youth in general will possess knowledge and skills that are appropriate for Aboriginal youth, particularly if such youth are living in urban environments or away from traditional territories. Moreover, as Chalmers et al. observed, those who wish to help Aboriginal youth should not be so focused on cultural awareness that they lose sight of the emotional needs that are clearly present.

Avoiding assumptions is another key point. Teachers and other professionals should consider the particular challenges that some Aboriginal youth may be facing, such as social problems due to discrimination, bullying, multiple deaths or losses among family and friends, or anger related to past injustices (Chalmers et al., 2014; Price & Dalgleish, 2013). At the same time, it is equally important that helpers not *assume* that a young person is facing any or all of these problems. As a research participant in Chalmers et al.'s (2014) study noted: "It is important to recognise historical factors that may lead to shame but essential that the first aider takes the adolescent on face value without pushing previous trauma upon them" (p. 8). It is also important to look for strengths and signs of resilience in youth; this emphasizes the positive aspects of MHL in contrast to a problem focus (Coverdale, Ambers, & Marshall, 2014).

Digital formats should be considered when working with adolescents. Today's digital youth spend significant amounts of time communicating online; this is also true for Aboriginal youth, particularly those in urban locations. As Kral (2014) observed, "communication via mobile phones and social networking has rapidly become the norm for Indigenous youth" (p. 171). Youth are comfortable online and can easily keep pace with new technologies that enable the revitalization of traditionally text-heavy materials into something they can access readily; for example, mental health information and resources can be transformed into digital visual formats such as websites, graphic novels, and videos (e.g., www.thehealthyaboriginal.net and www.youthbeyondblue.org). As some researchers have observed, online formats can be seen as more accessible and less threatening for hesitant help-seekers (Price & Dalgleish, 2013). The popularity of mobile phone apps, online chat services, and e-counselling among youth attest to the importance of using these new technologies in efforts to enhance youth MHL.

CONCLUSION

Many Aboriginal adolescents and young adults will continue to forgo beneficial and potentially life-saving mental health treatment unless help-seeking barriers such as access, cultural context, stigma, and lack of understanding are effectively addressed. A key strategy is to focus on adopting culturally relevant and culturally safe programs and practices to improve mental health literacy — both among the youth themselves as well as among the professionals who work with them. Schools, community youth programs, and youth-serving agencies offer developmentally appropriate learning and skill-building environments in which the promotion of MHL should be a priority. A central consideration is how to best actively engage and empower these youth in developmentally appropriate and culturally safe ways. To date, there is little information or evidence published about how teachers and educational programs can successfully foster MHL among Aboriginal youth; more research and evaluation studies are needed.

As Potvin-Boucher and Malone assert: "Our youth are our future and our responsibility" (2014, p. 344). A cultural approach is needed to foster mental health literacy among Aboriginal youth and the supporting adults who are working with them. In this chapter, several promising strategies, programs, and resources have been noted; most are readily adaptable to learning environments. Adopting a culturally relevant and culturally safe approach to MHL will benefit Aboriginal as well as non-Aboriginal youth and support them along the path of mental wellness.

Questions for Discussion, Reflection, and Writing

1. What do you know about local Aboriginal history and customs? How could you find out more?
2. Check one or more of the resources listed to support mental health literacy. How could you adapt them for use in your own classroom or professional setting?
3. Which of the points raised in "Fostering a climate for learning" would you find most challenging and how might you address that?

List of Online Resources

- Mental Health Commission of Canada – http://www.mental healthcommission.ca/English/issues/first-nations-inuit-and-metis
- Canadian Alliance on Mental Illness and Mental Health – http://www.camimh.ca/
- Beyond Blue – http://www.youthbeyondblue.com/

REFERENCES

Beyondblue. (2015). *Homepage.* Retrieved from www.beyondblue.org.au

Bourget, B. & Chenier, R. (2007). *Mental health literacy in Canada: Phase one report of the mental health literacy project.* Ottawa, ON: Canadian Alliance on Mental Illness and Mental Health.

Brascoupé, S. & Waters, C. (2009). Cultural safety exploring the applicability of the concept of cultural safety to Aboriginal health and community wellness. *International Journal of Indigenous Health*, *5*(2), 6–41.

Caza, M. (2010). *Final report: Evaluation of the Mental Health First Aid training in First Nations communities in Alberta.* Retrieved from http://www.mentalhealthfirstaid.ca/EN/about/Documents/Health_Canada_MHFA%20Evaluation%202010.pdf

Center for Native American Youth. (n.d.). *Fast facts on Native American youth and Indian country.* Washington, DC: Aspen Institute. Retrieved from http://www.aspeninstitute.org/sites/default/files/content/upload/ Native%20Youth%20Fast%20Facts%20Update_04-2014.pdf

Chalmers, K. J., Bond, K. S., Jorm, A. F., Kelly, C. M., Kitchener, B. A. & Williams-Tchen, A. J. (2014). Providing culturally appropriate mental health first aid to an Aboriginal or Torres Strait Islander adolescent: Development of expert consensus guidelines. *International Journal of Mental Health Systems*, *8*, 6–16.

Chandler, M. J. & Lalonde, C. E. (2008). Cultural continuity as a protective factor against suicide in First Nations youth. *Horizons – A Special Issue on Aboriginal Youth, Hope or Heartbreak: Aboriginal Youth and Canada's Future. 10*(1), 68–72.

Coverdale, J., Ambers, S. & Marshall, E. A. (2014, May). *"Stronger Together" – A community-university research partnership to support Indigenous youth identity and traditional knowledge*. Presentation at the CUVIC Conference on Beyond Engagement, University of Victoria, British Columbia, Canada.

First Nations Health Council. (2003). *Healthy children, healthy families, healthy communities: The road to wellness. British Columbia First Nations regional longitudinal health survey 2002/2003.* Retrieved from http://www.fnhc.ca/pdf/RHS_2002_2003_Regional_Report.pdf

Ganshorn, H. & Michaud, N. (2012). *Mental health first aid: An evidence review.* Calgary, AB: Mental Health Commission of Canada. Retrieved from http://www.mentalhealthfirstaid.ca/EN/about/Documents/MHFA%20Evidence%20Review%202012.pdf

Health Canada. (2011). *A statistical profile on the health of First Nations in Canada: Vital statistics for Atlantic and Western Canada, 2001/2002.* Ottawa, ON: Author. Retrieved from http://www.hc-sc.gc.ca/fniah-spnia/pubs/aborig-autoch/stats-profil-atlant/index-eng.php

Healthy Aboriginal Network. (2014). *Homepage.* Retrieved from http://thehealthyaboriginal.net/

Jorm, A. F. (2000). Mental health literacy: Public knowledge and beliefs about mental disorders. *British Journal of Psychiatry*, *177*, 396–401.

Jorm, A. F., Christensen, H. & Griffiths, K. M. (2005). Public beliefs about causes and risk factors for mental disorders: Changes in Australia over 8 years. *Social Psychiatry and Psychiatric Epidemiology*, *40*, 764–767.

Jorm, A. F., Korten, A. E., Jacomb, P. A., Christensen, H., Rodgers, B. & Pollitt, P. (1997). "Mental health literacy:" A survey of the public's ability to recognise mental disorders and their beliefs about the effectiveness of treatment. *Medical Journal of Australia*, *166*, 182–186.

Jorm, A. F., Morgan, A. J. & Wright, A. (2008). Interventions that are helpful for depression and anxiety in young people: A comparison of clinicians' beliefs with those of youth and their parents. *Journal of Affective Disorders*, *111*, 227–234.

Kanowski, L. G., Jorm, A. F. & Hart, L. M. (2009). A mental health first aid training program for Australian Aboriginal and Torres Strait Islander peoples: Description and initial evaluation. *International Journal of Mental Health Systems*, *3*(10). doi:10.1186/1752-4458-3-10.

Kelly, C. M., Mithen, J. M., Fischer, J. A., Kitchener, B. A., Jorm, A. F., Lowe, A. & Scanlan, C. (2011). Youth mental health first aid: A description of the program and an initial evaluation. *International Journal of Mental Health Systems*, *5*(4). doi:10.1186/1752-4458-5-4.

Kirmayer, L., Simpson, C. & Cargo, M. (2003). Healing traditions: Culture, community and mental health promotion with Canadian Aboriginal peoples. *Australasian Psychiatry*, *11*(1), s15–s23.

Kitchener, B. A. & Jorm, A. F. (2008). Mental Health First Aid: An international programme for early intervention. *Early Intervention in Psychiatry*, *2*, 55–61.

Kral, I. (2014). Shifting perception, shifting identities: Communication technologies and the altered social, cultural and linguistic ecology in a remote Indigenous context. *Australian Journal of Anthropology*, *25*, 171–189.

Lopes, J., Lindeman, M., Taylor, K. & Grant, L. (2012). Cross cultural education in suicide prevention: Development of a training resource for use in Central Australian Indigenous communities. *Australian E-journal for the Advancement of Mental Health*, *10*(3), 224–234.

Marcus, M. & Westra, H. (2012). Mental health literacy in Canadian young adults: Results of a national survey. *Canadian Journal of Community Mental Health*, *31*(1), 1–15.

Marshall, E. A., Coverdale, J. C., Roche, P. L., Lychowyd, L., Ramirez, P., Delaronde, L. & Cumming, J. (2014). *Aboriginal child & youth mental health: Practitioners' experiences of effective cultural support and treatment*. Unpublished manuscript, Centre for Youth & Society, University of Victoria, British Columbia, Canada. Available from http://www.youth.society.uvic.ca

McCarthy, J., Bruno, M. & Fernandes, T. E. (2011). Evaluating mental health literacy and adolescent depression: What do teenagers "know"? *The Professional Counselor. Research and Practice*, *1*(2), 133–142.

Mood Disorders Society of Canada. (2009). *Quick facts: Mental illness and addictions in Canada* (3rd ed.). Guelph, ON: Author. Retrieved from http://www.mooddisorderscanada.ca/page/quick-facts

Morrison, W. & Peterson, P. (2015). *Positive mental health toolkit*. Summerside, PE: Pan-Canadian Joint Consortium for School Health. Retrieved from http://www.jcshpositivementalhealthtoolkit.com/

Moses, T. (2010). Being treated differently: Stigma experiences with family, peers, and school staff among adolescents with mental health disorders. *Social Science and Medicine*, *70*(7), 985–993.

Nagel, T. M., Thompson, C., Robinson, G., Condon, J. & Trauer, T. (2009). Two-way approaches to Indigenous mental health literacy. *Australian Journal of Primary Health*, *15*(1), 50–55.

National Alliance on Mental Illness. (n.d.). *In our own voice*. Arlington, VA: Author.

Nuttgens, S. A. & Campbell, A. J. (2010). Multicultural considerations for counselling First Nations clients. *Canadian Journal of Counselling and Psychotherapy*, *44*(2), 115–129.

Pinfold, V., Stuart, H., Thornicroft, G. & Arboleda-Flórez, J. (2005). Working with young people: The impact of mental health awareness programmes in schools in the UK and Canada. *World Psychiatry*, *4*(1), 48–52.

Pinto-Foltz, M. D., Logsdon, M. C. & Myers, J. A. (2011). Feasibility, acceptability, and initial efficacy of a knowledge-contact program to reduce mental illness stigma and improve mental health literacy in adolescents. *Social Science & Medicine*, *72*, 2011–2019.

Potvin-Boucher, J. T. & Malone, J. L. (2014). Facilitating mental health literacy: Targeting Canadian First Nations youth. *Canadian Journal of Counselling and Psychotherapy*, *48*(3), 343–355.

Price, M. & Dalgleish, J. (2013). Help-seeking among Indigenous Australian adolescents. Exploring attitudes, behaviours and barriers. *Youth Studies Australia*, *32*(1), 10–18.

Public Health Agency of Canada. (2006). *The human face of mental health and mental illness in Canada 2006.* Ottawa, ON: Author. Retrieved from http://www.phac-aspc.gc.ca/publicat/human-humain06/index-eng.php

Ramsden, I. (1990). *Kawa whakaruruhau: Cultural safety in nursing education in Aotearoa.* Wellington, New Zealand: Ministry of Education.

Reavley, N. J. & Jorm, A. F. (2011a). *National survey of mental health literacy and stigma.* Canberra, Australia: Department of Health and Ageing.

Reavley, N. J. & Jorm, A. F. (2011b). Young people's recognition of mental disorders and beliefs about treatment and outcome: Findings from an Australian national survey. *Australian and New Zealand Journal of Psychiatry*, *45*, 890–898.

Smye, V., Browne, A. & Josewski, V. (2010). *Supporting the mental wellness of First Nations, Inuit and Métis peoples in Canada. Cultural safety: A research discussion paper* (A report for the Mood Disorders Society of Canada and the Native Mental Health Association of Canada). Available from the Native Mental Health Association of Canada, Chilliwack, BC.

Statistics Canada. (2013a). *Aboriginal Peoples in Canada: First Nations People, Métis and Inuit: The national household survey, 2011.* Ottawa, ON: Author. Retrieved from http://www12.statcan.gc.ca/nhs-enm/2011/ as-sa/99-011-x/99-011-x2011001-eng.cfm

Statistics Canada. (2013b). *Canada's total population estimates, 2013*. Ottawa, ON: Author. Retrieved from http://www.statcan.gc.ca/daily-quotidien/ 130926/dq130926a-eng.htm

Thira, D. (2014). Aboriginal youth suicide prevention: A post-colonial community-based approach. *International Journal of Child, Youth, & Family Studies*, *5*(1), 158–179.

United States Census Bureau. (2012). *The American Indian and Alaska Native population: 2010* (2010 Census Briefs). Washington, DC: Author. Retrieved from http://www.census.gov/prod/cen2010/briefs/c2010br-10.pdf

Westerman, T. (2010). Engaging Australian Aboriginal youth in mental health services. *Australian Psychologist*, *45*(3), 212–222.

Whitley, J., Smith, J. D. & Vaillancourt, T. (2013). Promoting mental health literacy among educators: Critical in school-based prevention and intervention. *Canadian Journal of School Psychology*, *28*(1), 56–70.

Wile Schwarz, S. (2009). *Adolescent mental health in the United States: Facts for policymakers.* New York, NY: Columbia University & National Center for Children in Poverty. Retrieved from http://www.nccp. org/publications/pub_878.html

youthbeyondblue. (2015). *Homepage.* Retrieved from www.youthbeyondblue.com

In: Adolescent Health Literacy and Learning
Editors: D. L. Begoray and E. M. Banister
ISBN: 978-1-63482-897-0

Chapter 8

MENTAL HEALTH LITERACIES IN YOUTH WORK PRACTICE WITH ADOLESCENTS

Patti Ranahan*
Department of Applied Human Sciences, Concordia University, Canada

ABSTRACT

While the concept of health literacy has undergone transformations and additions since its conception, the definition of mental health literacy has remained close to its original form. Informed by critical and social literacy theories and recent research examining youth work practice with suicidal adolescents, the author offers a re-envisioned definition of mental health literacy. This fresh definition recognizes literacy as a relational and contextualized social practice and identifies previously omitted knowledges and skills in current notions of literacy in mental health. Broadening our understanding of what constitutes literacy unlocks new possibilities for responding to adolescents impacted by mental health and suicide concerns.

Keywords: mental health literacy, youth work, critical literacy, social literacy, suicide intervention

INTRODUCTION

Focusing Questions

1. Why is mental health literacy important in youth work practice?
2. How might current conceptualizations of mental health literacy be re-envisioned for youth work practice with suicidal adolescents?

* Corresponding author (email): Patti.Ranahan@concordia.ca.

Youth work practice is dynamic, flexible, creative, and complex (Harland & Morgan, 2006). The complexities of youth work are compounded in situations involving suicide. White (2012) described youth suicide as "a 'wild' and unruly problem that is deeply embedded in local, historical, political and relational contexts" (p. 42) and that cannot be resolved through standardized approaches or application of specific procedures. As such, it is suggested in this chapter that current conceptualizations of mental health literacy may not serve youth work practice and, specifically, youth work practice with suicidal adolescents. The concept must be re-envisioned and developed further to include presently unarticulated literacies required for these intricate interventions with young people.

While the concept of health literacy has undergone numerous developments, additions, and transformations since its definition by Simonds in 1974 (Rootman, Frankish, & Kaszap, 2007), mental health literacy continues to be defined in ways close to its original form. Jorm et al. (1997) initially defined the concept of mental health literacy as "knowledge and beliefs about mental disorders which aid their recognition, management or prevention" (p. 182). The Canadian Alliance on Mental Illness and Mental Health (2008) included the ability to "access, understand and apply information" and focused on empowerment of individuals in making informed decisions to promote mental health (p. 5). Currently, the concept is applied in mental health literacy research from a traditional notion of literacy whereby literacy is viewed as located within individual persons and centres on the ability to read and write (Norton, 2007). That is, people are deemed illiterate (i.e., unskilled) or literate (i.e., intelligent and civilized; Gee, 2007; Street, 2009), and literacy is viewed as measurable and as attributable to individuals (Scribner, 1984; Street, 1995). Research methods designed to examine literacy in mental health primarily rely on large cross-sectional surveys that are used to test individuals' declared knowledge of mental disorders (e.g., knowledge of the signs of major depression) or knowledge of treatments available for specific mental disorders (Goldney, Fisher, & Wilson, 2001; Olsson & Kennedy, 2010; Wang et al., 2007). Research conducted with such methods "rips literacy out of its sociocultural contexts and treats it as a social cognitive skill with little or nothing to do with human relationships" (Gee, 2007, p. 67). Now is the time to re-imagine mental health literacy as a situated, contextualized social practice requiring knowledges and skills that are immeasurable, unquantifiable, and enhanced through experience by means of innovative and creative methods.

In this chapter, the traditional notion of mental health literacy is challenged for the purpose of extending our comprehension of what knowledges, skills, understandings, and/or experiences are relevant for youth work practice with suicidal adolescents. First, an overview of literacy theories, including critical literacy theory and social literacy theory, that are pertinent to my purpose of re-imagining what mental health literacy may entail is provided. Secondly, the complexities of youth work practice with young people who are suicidal and draw upon recent research and scholarly literature that has identified additional knowledges and skills required for mental health literacy for youth workers are discussed. Woven into this section is the story of a youth worker, named *Alice*, who encounters a young person, *Antoine*, who is contemplating ending his life. Lastly, a re-envisioned conceptualization of mental health literacy that incorporates the theoretical constructs of literacy reviewed in the initial section and responds to the complexities of youth work practice with suicidal adolescents is offered. In closing, Alice and Antoine's story returns and, in concrete and practical terms, this new vision of mental health literacy for youth work practice with young people is operationalized.

CRITICAL AND SOCIAL LITERACY THEORETICAL CONSTRUCTS

Re-envisioning the concept of mental health literacy requires exploration of *literacy* itself. Kirsch (2001) described literacy as being comprised of cumulative skills, knowledges, and strategies that individuals acquire during their lives via their participation in interactions, contexts, and communities. It is "inherently situated in personal, historical, cultural, and social contexts" (Cervetti, Damico, & Pearson, 2006, p. 380) and "encompasses any form of communication" (Wood, 2002, p. 1). Further, literacy may be understood as a social construction and social practice (Menezes de Souza, 2007). Bearing such conceptions of literacy in mind, this section presents a brief overview of critical literacy theory and social literacy theory to set the stage for reconceptualizing what literacy in mental health may involve for youth work practice.

Critical Literacy

Critical literacy involves a process comprised of three features: empowerment, awareness leading to transformation, and social action. Empowerment acknowledges that power is located within particular roles (e.g., teacher/student) and attempts to shift the power within these roles (e.g., through a redefinition of roles). Redefining roles requires those with power to relinquish their power (McDaniel, 2004) and engage in collaborative knowledge making (Gee, 2007) where the creation of knowledge is a "relational act" (Giroux, 1987, p. 15). Empowerment requires a learning environment that promotes learners' sense of agency, self-sufficiency, and confidence (McDaniel, 2004).

Empowerment leads to awareness as learners are able to participate fully, critically question, and collaborate with others in the learning environment. Through a shifting of roles and increased awareness, learners are transformed through understanding their own capacity to transform their lives (Freire, 1970). As learners are empowered to question, participate, and value their own experiences and knowledge, they become conscious of the realities of their lives and those around them and are called to social action. This action consists of addressing inequities, promoting justice, and challenging the status quo (Shor, 1999). That is, critical literacy theory includes "learning how to interpret and act on the world in socially just ways" (Kendrick, Rogers, Smythe, & Anderson, 2005, p. 2) along with a duty to work toward change (McDaniel, 2004).

Empowerment, awareness and transformation, and social action are key characteristics of critical literacy theory that challenge the notion of literacy as being located within individuals or as a measurable, fixed attribute. Further, characteristics of empowerment and awareness invite a unique level of participation in defining *what* constitutes knowledge(s) and summons critical reflection on *who* defines the knowledge(s) to be known. For example, in their early definition, Jorm et al. (1997) suggested that knowledge of mental disorders is a key feature of mental health literacy. Mental health literacy research has traditionally focused on examining populations' abilities to identify mental disorders (e.g., depression) according to the *Diagnostic and Statistical Manual of Mental Health Disorders* (DSM; American Psychiatric Association, 2013). Applying literacy in mental health from a critical literacy approach would include shifting the balance of power away from the DSM criteria for diagnosis of mental disorders by inviting people to self-identify what the challenge is and how it impacts their functioning and wellbeing. Additionally, people would be encouraged to participate in a collaborative fashion to establish a process for alleviating their struggle.

Social Literacy Theory

Social literacy theorists challenge the notion of literacy in two ways: first, as a measurable attribute that is acquired through schooling and, second, as a complex social practice (Ivanic, 2009; New London Group [NLG], 2000). Literacy does not have a universal essence that can be captured (Scribner, 1984) because it is contextually situated within interactions and relationships (Street, 1995). Literacy is influenced by and created by the social context, the individuals involved and their actions, and the activities in which they engage (Prinsloo & Baynham, 2008). That is, there are variances of literacy from one context to another and the uses and meanings people bring to the context (Street, 2009).

As a social practice, multiple literacies may be required for a particular context (Ivanic, 2009); yet it is not enough to simply offer a list of competencies for a particular situation to deem individuals literate or illiterate. Additionally, it is not sufficient to impart standardized one-size-fits-all procedures for interventions that require persons to enact literacy practices. A pluralistic view of literacy considers "the complexity of meaning making" individuals undertake within a particular context that includes conditions of power, identities, or culture (Street, 2009, p. 26).

Literacy acquisition in social literacy theory is a process whereby learners engage critically with the content and material and connect to experience (NLG, 2000). Innovation and creativity are emphasized in the learning process (NLG, 2000), and the focus is on apprenticeship or experiences that are built upon, rather than acquired (Gee, 2010). As such, social literacy theorists would suggest literacy in mental health is garnered through evolving experiences and located in interactions. A youth worker's encounter with a young person who is suicidal may be a site for learning and enhancing literacy in mental health, yet it is also a site that is contextually situated with unique conditions influencing the interaction. For example, the young person's cultural background and beliefs about suicide or the specific organizational policy that the youth worker's employer provides impact the youth worker's literacy in mental health during the interaction. Recently, scholars have begun to recognize the influence of conditions, such as cultural perspectives on literacy in mental health, and have challenged notions of standardized educational approaches to suicide intervention that tend to neglect the situatedness of the interaction (Wexler, White, & Trainor, 2015). Suicide must be viewed as a problem that has political, relational, social, historical, or cultural dimensions and not solely as an individual problem (Wexler & Gone, 2012). However, the intersections of context, culture, communication, technology, or confounders are not taken up in current health literacy research (Mancuso, 2008) or considered in current mental health literacy educational interventions.

Social and critical literacy theorists view literacy as a relational act and set of social practices (Barton & Hamilton, 2000; Street, 1995, 2009) that are comprised of activities, actions, and interactions within a specified context (Prinsloo & Baynham, 2008). This review of critical and social literacy theories provides the theoretical basis and rationale for re-imagining a definition for mental health literacy. The complexities of youth work practice, and specifically the challenge of practice with suicidal adolescents, add to this call for extending what constitutes literacy in mental health.

YOUTH WORK PRACTICE WITH SUICIDAL ADOLESCENTS

Promoting the optimal development of young people through informal education, collaborative and voluntary relationships, creating environments, and responding flexibly to young people's needs are some of the key features of youth work practice (Davies, 2010; Freeman, 2013; Harland & Morgan, 2006; Merton, 2004; Spence, 2008). Youth work practice (also referred to as child and youth care practice) occurs in the everyday lives or *lifespace* of young people (Gharabaghi & Stuart, 2011); youth workers may engage with young people in a range of settings including child welfare, residential group care, schools, hospitals, or community-based contexts. As the first onset of many mental health concerns occurs in childhood or adolescence (Kessler et al., 2007) and adolescents are in a higher risk group for suicide (Pelkonen & Marttunen, 2003; Shaw, Fernandes, & Rao, 2005), it is likely that youth workers will encounter young people experiencing mental health concerns and/or suicidality throughout their career.

The following story of a youth worker and a 16-year-old is provided to illustrate the complexities of youth work practice with suicidal adolescents. Details of the story are derived from the author's interviews with multiple youth workers and prior youth work experience with young people. Names and identifying information have been changed.

> Anna is a youth worker in a group home for six adolescents in a large urban centre. As a recent graduate of an undergraduate program in youth work studies, despite the shift-work requirement to work evenings and weekends, Anna welcomed the opportunity to gain practice experience in a residential care setting. She arrived one Sunday evening for her shift and began to read the communication log — a record of the daily events for each resident recorded by the youth workers on the previous shift. Anna read the brief background information provided about the new resident, Antoine, who arrived at the group home that morning. According to the log, 16-year-old Antoine was placed in the group home after he attempted suicide by hanging in the foster home where he had resided for the past 10 years. He was not to return to the foster home, and the auxiliary social worker who placed him in the group home indicated he would likely be eligible for the independent living program. The social worker directed that Antoine be placed on a suicide watch whereby the youth workers would observe Antoine and keep him within arms' length. Anna felt somewhat panicked when she read about Antoine's suicidality as this was her first encounter with this issue in practice. She had attended a workshop on suicide intervention during her undergraduate degree but believed that she was unprepared for this situation.
>
> Antoine was watching television by himself when Anna arrived. The other residents of the group home were in the community visiting friends or family members. Anna approached Antoine and tried to engage him in conversation. He was talkative, and they started playing a game of pool. During the game, Antoine turned to Anna and said, "I'm here 'cause I tried to hang myself you know. It freaked out my foster parents and now they don't want me back. So now I got nobody and might as well just off myself." Anna felt a lump in her throat. She didn't know how to respond! She remembered from the

> workshop that she was supposed to ask directly if he was thinking of suicide, but he had already told her he was thinking of killing himself. So what should she say now? Anna knew from what she had read in her youth studies program that adolescents as a group were at higher risk for suicide, that hanging was the most common method used, that males die by suicide more often than females as they are likely to choose more lethal means, and that children in child welfare settings were also a high-risk group. She also knew that the phone number for emergency mental health services was in the staff office and that the suicide protocol at the group home required her to notify her supervisor and the youth's social worker immediately if a youth was suicidal. Anna took a deep breath, looked at Antoine, and saw he was hurting. He was waiting for her to respond, waiting for her to engage, and waiting for her to be present and connected with him in his psychological pain. Just as she turned to respond with empathy, caring, and relational presence, she paused. Her mind raced with questions. What would happen to her job if she didn't follow the protocol and immediately inform her supervisor? Would she be terminated from her position? What if he killed himself on her shift? Would she be responsible?

Like many youth workers, Anna participated in educational workshops on suicide intervention that had provided her with information regarding risk factors and coached her on asking directly about suicide. Generally, mental health content in preservice education is quite limited (Ranahan, 2013a); recent research on youth work practice suggests that literacy in mental health involves knowledges not currently taken up in contemporary views of mental health literacy (Ranahan, 2013b, 2014) or in mental health and suicide education. Knowledge of risk factors may be beneficial in identifying groups to target for prevention activities; however, this knowledge has limited practical usefulness in the moment between Anna and Antoine illustrated above. The following section provides a review of research findings that suggest new understandings of how literacy may be developed and what literacy in mental health may entail for youth workers.

Youth Workers' Development of Mental Health Literacy

As noted previously, traditional approaches to literacy acquisition have focused on schooling or education programs. Such traditional approaches to mental health literacy development are rampant especially for the topic of suicide. Youth workers are exposed to brief educational events, often referred to as gatekeeper training, as a means of teaching youth workers about the warning signs of suicidality or mental health disorders and enhancing the knowledge of available mental health services (Burns & Patton, 2000). The role of a youth worker has been defined as a *gatekeeper* in the literature (Bourke & Evans, 2000; Rickwood, Deane, & Wilson, 2007) whereby youth workers are able to identify a young person at risk for suicide and initiate a referral to services that provide mental health care. Training programs such as Mental Health First Aid (Jorm, Kitchener, Kanowski, & Kelly, 2007) and Applied Suicide Intervention Skills Training (LivingWorks Education, 2007) are offered to youth workers as short educational interventions to enhance literacy in mental health and suicide. Despite the popularity of these traditional approaches to literacy acquisition, recent research suggests youth workers' mental health literacy is more powerfully developed through practical experience and best viewed as an evolving process.

Ranahan and Pellissier's (2015) discourse analysis of youth workers' talk of their experiences with suicidal young people revealed the importance of the first encounter with a situation involving suicide to their literacy development. In the study, three youth workers who had encountered a young person who was suicidal participated in an audio- and video-recorded conversation. These youth workers spontaneously chose to share the story of their first experience with a suicidal youth and discursively constructed this experience as a two-dimensional process of moving from not knowing to knowing, that is, crossing a knowledge barrier. Additionally, their first experience endured over time as they held fast to such stories throughout their career. Ranahan and Pellissier posited that these experiences were discursively constructed as "touchstones, or familiar stories" — a term Strong-Wilson (2006, p. 61) applied to stories that are formative in regard to a practitioner's sense of self and to which all future experiences are compared. Further, Strong-Wilson suggested these stories cannot be erased or changed, thereby highlighting the power of initial experiences in practice with adolescents experiencing suicidality in a youth worker's learning and development of mental health literacy.

Considering this recent research, approaches to enhancing literacy in mental health for youth workers must be re-evaluated. As critical literacy theorists suggest, pedagogical approaches to enhancing literacy are well suited for learning activities that are focused on transforming thinking instead of teaching technical skills (McDaniel, 2004). Literacy development is a process of reflection (Mayo, 2004) where learners critique, question, and evaluate the assumptions embedded within a curriculum (McDaniel, 2004). Social literacy theorists emphasize apprenticeship over acquisition, suggesting that mental health literacy development is a relational and interactional process (NLG, 2000). Youth workers' initial practical experiences, such as Anna's encounter with Antoine, are foundational to learning and professional development and are rich opportunities for mentorship, supervision, and guidance in the enhancement of knowledges for practice with young people experiencing mental health concerns.

Features of Literacy in Mental Health for Youth Workers

Research examining child and youth care professionals' mental health literacies in encounters with suicidal adolescents illuminated new literacies needed for effective youth work practice with young people experiencing mental health concerns that are not included in the current conceptualization. For example, literacies in mental health for youth workers include relational knowledges. Ranahan (2013a) identified the literacy practice of *being with* an adolescent who is contemplating ending his/her life. Being with involves relational knowing whereby the youth worker is able to be present and attentive to the young person and to engage in a collaborative manner. Being with includes nonverbal communication as professionals express energetically through a physical presence their connection to the adolescent. Professionals described empathic caring about the young person and the psychological pain they were experiencing. Returning to the illustration above, Anna could draw upon her skills in communicating empathy and being present and fully engaged with Antoine by inviting him to share more about his experience. The knowledges of risk factors or protocols may, in the initial moments of this suicide intervention, distract from Anna's ability to engage relationally with Antoine and may impede her ability to practice effectively (i.e., remain relationally engaged with Antoine). Thus, in youth work practice, literacy in mental health must include relational knowledges and skills in collaboration, empathic verbal and non-verbal communication, and a caring approach when meeting the needs of young people experiencing mental health concerns.

Mental health literacy for youth workers additionally includes knowledge of the larger mental health system of care and skills in developing cooperative partnerships with other services. The current conceptualization of mental health literacy encompasses knowledge of services available (Jorm et al., 1997); however, for youth workers, this feature of literacy requires additional attention. Ranahan (2013c) identified the literacy practice of referring young people to other mental health service providers as *flooding the zone*. Upon learning of a young person's thoughts of suicide or suicidal behavior, the professional would contact other service providers to surround the adolescent with mental health professionals who may be known or unknown to the adolescent. Often this process would situate the youth worker on the periphery or at a physical distance from the young person, thus fracturing his/her ability to be physically attentive and engaged within the youth worker–youth relational connection even when the youth wanted to receive care from the youth worker. For example, if Anna left Antoine to immediately inform her supervisor and his social worker of his thoughts of suicide, her engagement with him would be interrupted; and it is likely that his willingness to collaborate with her in maintaining safety may be compromised. Thus, literacy in mental health for youth workers includes maintaining a relational connection with the young person and *being with* — all while knowing what services are available, how to access the services (including knowledge of strategies to expedite access), and skills in negotiation, advocacy, and communication in order to effectively navigate the mental health system.

Literacy in mental health for youth work practice also involves the knowledge and ability to critically examine current systems and policies that support potentially oppressive practices and/or limit possibilities for supportive mental health care. Employers often supply policies to youth workers or other helping professionals that outline procedures for responding to young people experiencing suicidality. To illustrate, observational practices are used to monitor the safety of suicidal individuals, such as the monitoring of Antoine in the group home. Such practices may be referred to as a suicide watch (Junker, Beeler, & Bates, 2005; Ranahan, 2014) or constant observation (Alland, Gallagher, & Henderson, 2003). Procedurally, a suicide watch involves professionals surveying the suicidal person through direct observation at regular intervals, monitoring via surveillance cameras, maintaining the person in line of sight, and documenting the practice (Clinical Resource & Audit Group, 2002; Junker et al., 2005; Ranahan, 2014). When policies meant to guide youth workers' practice were insufficient for the situation or appeared limited, practitioners relied on intuition or "gut feeling" to make decisions (Ranahan, 2014, p. 15). However, a reliance on gut feelings to guide practice is inadequate in the face of supporting young people experiencing mental health concerns and suicide where death and psychological suffering is at hand. Literacy in mental health for youth work must include the ability to challenge policies that may not meet the needs of an individual adolescent and to critically examine, question, and reflect on how policies impede or create opportunities in practice (Ranahan, 2014). In conversations with her supervisor or youth work colleagues, Anna could raise critical questions about the process of informing a young person's social worker or her supervisor. She may suggest the protocol be changed to explicitly include inviting youth workers to remain with the young person while therapeutically engaged and creating a space for collaboration with the youth in identifying who may be an additional support to talk to. Mental health literacy needs to include elements of empowerment where youth workers can challenge processes that impede or interrupt the relational therapeutic process with young people while still maintaining the importance of accountability.

The summary of recent research on youth work interventions with young people at risk for suicide provided above suggests that the current conceptualization of mental health literacy is inadequate for youth work practice and the concept needs to be re-imagined to include additional knowledges and skills that are not currently articulated (Ranahan, 2013a, 2013c, 2014). Youth workers can develop literacy in mental health through profound experiences in practice and not necessarily through a traditional schooling approach. Further, mental health literacy for youth workers includes relational knowledges that emphasize skills in engagement, empathy, collaboration, communication, and presence with youth who are psychologically suffering. Knowledge of mental health services or treatments available are insufficient for youth work practice because youth workers need to be able to negotiate and advocate in the mental health system of care — all while maintaining relational engagement with the young person. Critical reflection and challenging systems, structures, and policies that impede practice are important skills necessary for mental health literacy for youth workers. Thus, it is time to conceive of a new, more broadly defined conceptualization of mental health literacy, especially for youth work practice with suicidal young people.

Re-envisioning the Concept of Mental Health Literacy

Adolescents desire help for health and mental health concerns from those they have relationships with and from carers who are trusting, confidential, accepting, caring, supportive, and genuine (Bowers, Manion, Papadopoulos, & Gauvreau, 2012; Boyd et al., 2007; Guliver, Griffiths, & Christensen, 2010; Knighton & Currie, 2010; Purcell et al., 2011; Sheffield, Fiorenza, & Sofronoff, 2004; Wilson & Deane, 2001). Youth workers taking up the gatekeeper role and referring an adolescent to specialized mental health services may not be well-received by adolescents in their care as young people prefer help from those with whom they have an existing relationship (Ranahan, 2013c). From a critical literacy perspective, youth workers need to be empowered to question and examine dominant knowledges in mental health and participate fully in collaboration with young people, colleagues, and helpers across disciplines in providing suicide care. A social literacy perspective recognizes the social context as a location of mental health literacy construction and the participants in the interaction as co-constructors of collective mental health knowledge making. Research on youth workers' discursive constructions of mental health literacy and mental health literacy practices in encounters with suicidal adolescents suggests that initial experiences are central to literacy development and that there are multiple literacies involved in youth work practice with young people experiencing mental health concerns or suicide.

Upon consideration of the theories of social literacy and critical literacy, and the research outlining the complexities of youth work practice with suicidal adolescents, the following reconceptualization of mental health literacy is needed: collective knowledges, meanings, and experiences of mental health that aid in awareness (e.g., consciousness of conditions and sociocultural realities that shape lives) and transformation (e.g., conceptions of change, possibilities, optimism, hope) and that enable emancipatory action (e.g., access, availability of resources that are designed and desired by young people) and full participation (e.g., relational, collaborative, partnership in care) in maintaining and enhancing mental wellness across variable, localized contexts. Rather than being fixed or absolute, this definition is intended to spark further imagination and open up new possibilities for understanding mental health literacy in the context of youth suicide prevention practice and research. The re-envisioned definition unlocks fresh options in developing mental health literacy educational initiatives that go beyond a Western view of mental health, which can be very limiting (Joyce et al., 2011). Further, it allows for different kinds of knowledges to be considered in exploring what is *good* mental health literacy (Gladstone, 2010) and makes room for local and relational meaning making in interactions between professionals and young people (White & Morris, 2010). Future research could include inquiry into the interactional process of help-seeking (Cartmill, Deane, & Wilson, 2009) and changing the *ownership* of mental health care by identifying (in collaboration with young people) *who* can help (Kutcher, Davidson, & Manion, 2009; Mazzer, Rickwood, & Vanags, 2012). By re-envisioning the concept of mental health literacy, the intent is to follow White and Stoneman's (2012) suggestion:

> recommending ways of thinking and doing prevention that capitalize on young people's wisdom, recognize more collaborative approaches to knowledge-making and community building, and enable multiple forms of critical engagement and resistance as well as engendering practices of hope and solidarity. (p. 104)

If the current decontextualized conceptualization of mental health literacy continues to influence literacy education and research practices where efforts are continuously preoccupied with *correct* identification of mental disorders or measuring literacy levels within populations (Lam, 2014), this will impede the emergence of innovative, creative, and collaborative approaches to resolving the wild problem of youth suicide (White, 2012).

A Return to Anna and Antoine

The situation between Anna and Antoine unfolds further as an illustration of how the re-envisioned conceptual definition of mental health literacy may be operationalized in youth work practice with suicidal adolescents. Features of the new definition are indicated in brackets as the story unfolds.

> Anna turns her attention back to Antoine. She will discuss her questions about the suicide protocol with her youth work colleagues and supervisor at the staff meeting tomorrow [consciousness of the policy conditions that are shaping her interaction]. To ensure they both understand what Antoine is talking about [collective meanings], Anna asks him what he means in his statement "he might as well off himself." Antoine speaks at length with Anna openly about his thoughts of suicide, his feelings of isolation and abandonment by his foster family, and his hope that his foster parents will be able to have a relationship with him in the future even though he scared them with his suicide attempt.

> Anna asks Antoine what he would like to do this evening with Anna to help himself feel better [full participation]. Antoine states that he already feels better after talking with Anna [availability of resources that are designed and desired by young people] and discloses that he is an artist and loves to draw. Antoine asks Anna if she would help him send his artwork to his foster parents if he was to create a piece this evening. Anna agrees and, as she supports Antoine in setting up a place in the group home where he can draw, she reflects on the change in his emotional energy. She realizes her engagement with Antoine and his participation in deciding what would be helpful for him has her feeling more optimistic, and less fearful, about her work with Antoine and facing situations involving suicide in the future [transformation]. She leaves Antoine to engage in his art project and heads to the staff room to call her supervisor.

A key difference between the novice youth worker and the youth worker with expertise is the ability to consider the youth's context and identify a variety of responses for a particular situation (Larson, Rickman, Gibbons, & Walker, 2009). Bessant (2012) described youth work as "multi-faceted, dynamic, messy, and unpredictable work that requires expertise that cannot be rote learned by following rules or instructions" (p. 62). Anna's re-envisioned mental health literacies in the situation with Antoine illustrate a youth worker who can draw upon a variety of skills, identify a range of responses including eliciting Antoine's full participation in identifying what can help, and attend to the organization's policies in an accountable way. While she may not be able to recite the criteria for depression according to the DSM, she is responsive, engaged, and supporting Antoine's life and reasons for living. These features are significant for literacy in mental health in youth work practice with suicidal adolescents.

CONCLUSION

Problems such as suicide are wild and not easily solved with standardized approaches to intervention (White, 2012); they cannot be taught in educational endeavours via one-size-fits-all methods (Wexler et al., 2015). Adolescent suicide is a challenge for youth workers and other helping professionals; it is complex and a result of an intricate weaving of multiple factors. A conceptualization of literacy in mental health that does not acknowledge such complexities, or the wildness and situatedness of the problem of suicide (White, 2012), cannot adequately illuminate the knowledges and skills needed for effective youth work practice in situations involving suicide. Social literacy theory and critical literacy theory offer greater insight into how the present definition of mental health literacy may be broadened and re-imagined to include the knowledges and skills found in recent research examining youth work practice with suicidal adolescents. Relational knowledges, skills in collaborative practice, negotiation, critical thinking, advocacy, and the ability to challenge systemic and procedural constraints (e.g., access to mental health care, engagement in observational practices) can be integrated in a new vision of mental health literacy for youth work practice. Broadening what constitutes mental health literacy may permit youth workers to respond to young people in psychological distress with "strategies that emphasize multiplicity, interpretation, dialogue and negotiation instead of certainty and expert control" (White, 2012, p. 47). Such responses by youth workers may encourage young people like

Antoine to engage with life-giving activities and seek out support from others when they are feeling suicidal.

Questions for Discussion, Reflection, and Writing

1. Do you agree with the author that a new, re-envisioned definition of mental health literacy is needed? Why or why not?
2. Based on the new definition of mental health literacy offered in this chapter, how might current conceptualizations of health literacy be altered or extended?
3. After reading this chapter, has your view of what constitutes literacy changed or been challenged? If so, in what ways?

List of Online Resources

- Mind your Mind – mindyourmind.ca
- Mad in America: Science, Psychiatry and Community – madinamerica.com
- Teen Mental Health – teenmentalhealth.org

REFERENCES

Alland, C., Gallagher, A. & Henderson, J. (2003). Staying close: Creating distance? The ethics of constant observation. *Mental Health Practice*, *7*(3), 15–16.

American Psychiatric Association. (2013). *Diagnostic and statistical manual of mental health disorders* (5th ed.). Washington, DC: Author.

Barton, D. & Hamilton, M. (2000). Literacy practices. In D. Barton, M. Hamilton, & R. Ivanic (Eds.), *Situated literacies: Reading and writing in context* (pp. 7–15). New York, NY: Routledge.

Bessant, J. (2012). Youth work and the education of professional practitioners in Australia. In D. Fusco (Ed.), *Advancing youth work: Current trends, critical questions* (pp. 52–68). New York, NY: Routledge.

Bourke, L. & Evans, P. (2000). Youth workers in Sydney: Doing a lot with a little. *Youth Studies Australia*, *19*(1), 38–43.

Bowers, H., Manion, I., Papadopoulos, D. & Gauvreau, E. (2012). Stigma in school-based mental health: Perceptions of young people and service providers. *Child and Adolescent Mental Health*, *18*(3), 165–170.

Boyd, C., Francis, K., Aisbett, D., Newnham, K., Sewell, J., Dawes, G. & Nurse, S. (2007). Australian rural adolescents' experiences of accessing psychological help for a mental health problem. *Australian Journal of Rural Health*, *15*, 196–200.

Burns, J. M. & Patton, G. C. (2000). Preventive interventions for youth suicide: A risk factor-based approach. *Australian and New Zealand Journal of Psychiatry*, *34*, 388–407.

Canadian Alliance on Mental Illness and Mental Health. (2008). *National integrated framework for enhancing mental health literacy in Canada*. Retrieved from http://www.mooddisorderscanada.ca/documents/Publications/CAMIMH%20National%20Integrated%20Framework%20for%20Mental%20Health%20Literacy.pdf

Cartmill, T., Deane, F. P. & Wilson, C. J. (2009). Gatekeeper training for youth workers: Impact on mental health help-seeking and referral skill. *Youth Studies Australia, 28*(1), 5–12.

Cervetti, G., Damico, J. & Pearson, D. P. (2006). Multiple literacies, new literacies, and teacher education. *Theory into Practice, 45*(4), 296–303.

Clinical Resource & Audit Group. (2002). *Engaging people. Observation of people with acute mental health problems: A good practice statement.* Edinburgh, Scotland: Stationary Office Bookshop. Retrieved from http://www.scotland.gov.uk/Resource/Doc/46951/0013967.pdf

Davies, B. (2010). What do we mean by youth work? In J. Batsleer & B. Davies (Eds.), *What is youth work?* (pp. 1–6). Exeter, England: Learning Matters.

Freeman, J. (2013). The field of child and youth care: Are we there yet? *Child & Youth Services, 34*(2), 100–111.

Freire, P. (1970). The adult literacy process as cultural action for freedom. *Harvard Educational Review, 40*(2), 205–225.

Gee, J. P. (2007). *Social linguistics and literacies: Ideology in discourses* (3rd ed.). New York, NY: Routledge.

Gee, J. P. (2010). A situated-sociocultural approach to literacy and technology. In E. A. Baker (Ed.), *The new literacies: Multiple perspectives on research and practice* (pp. 165–193). New York, NY: Guilford Press.

Gharabaghi, K. & Stuart, C. (2011). *Right here, right now: Exploring life-space interventions for children and youth.* Toronto, ON: Pearson Education.

Giroux, H. A. (1987). Introduction: Literacy and the pedagogy of political empowerment. In P. Freire & D. Macedo (Eds.), *Literacy: Reading the world and the word* (pp. 1–25). South Hadley, MA: Bergin and Garvey.

Gladstone, B. M. (2010). *"All in the same boat": An analysis of a support group for children of parents with mental illnesses* (Doctoral dissertation). Retrieved from ProQuest Dissertations & Theses A&I. (870508607)

Goldney, R. D., Fisher, L. J. & Wilson, D. H. (2001). Mental health literacy: An impediment to the optimum treatment of major depression in the community. *Journal of Affective Disorders, 64*, 277–284.

Guliver, A., Griffiths, K. M. & Christensen, H. (2010). Perceived barriers and facilitators to mental health help-seeking in young people: A systematic review. *BMC Psychiatry, 10*, 113. doi:10.1186/1471-244X-10-113

Harland, K. & Morgan, T. (2006). Youth work in Northern Ireland: An exploration of emerging themes and challenges. *Youth Studies Ireland, 1*(1), 4–18.

Ivanic, R. (2009). Bringing literacy studies into research on learning across the curriculum. In M. Baynham & M. Prinsloo (Eds.), *The future of literacy studies* (pp. 100–122). New York, NY: Palgrave Macmillan.

Jorm, A. F., Kitchener, B. A., Kanowski, L. G. & Kelly, C. M. (2007). Mental health first aid training for members of the public. *International Journal of Clinical and Health Psychology, 7*, 141–151.

Jorm, A. F., Korten, A. E., Jacomb, P. A., Christensen, H., Rodgers, B. & Pollitt, P. (1997). "Mental health literacy": A survey of the public's ability to recognise mental disorders and their beliefs about the effectiveness of treatment. *Medical Journal of Australia*, *166*, 182–186.

Joyce, T., Higgins, I., Magin, P., Goode, S., Pond, D., Stone, T. … O'Neill, K. (2011). Nurses' perceptions of a mental health education programme for Australian nurses. *International Journal of Mental Health Nursing*, *20*, 247–252.

Junker, G., Beeler, A. & Bates, J. (2005). Using trained inmate observers for suicide watch in a federal correctional setting: A win-win solution. *Psychological Services*, *2*(1), 20–27.

Kendrick, M., Rogers, T., Smythe, S. & Anderson, J. (2005). Portraits of literacy across families, communities, and schools: An introduction. In J. Anderson, M. Kendrick, T. Rogers, & S. Smythe (Eds.), *Portraits of literacy across families, communities, and schools: Intersections and tensions* (1–20). Mahwah, NJ: Lawrence Erlbaum.

Kessler, R. C., Amminger, G. P., Aguilar Gaxiola, S., Alonso, J., Lee, S. & Ustun, T. B. (2007). Age of onset of mental disorders: A review of recent literature. *Current Opinion in Psychiatry*, *20*(4), 359–364.

Kirsch, I. (2001, December). *The international adult learning survey: Understanding what was measured*. Retrieved from https://www.ets.org/ Media/ Research/ pdf/RR-01-25-Kirsch.pdf

Knighton, L. & Currie, J. (2010). *Mental health literacy: Kids in Canada talk about mental health* (Kids Help Phone Critical Issue Report). Retrieved from http://events.kidshelpphone.ca/ flipbooks/Mental_Health_Full/files/ cir2010-en-final.pdf

Kutcher, S., Davidson, S. & Manion, I. (2009). Child and youth mental health: Integrated health care using contemporary competency-based teams. *Pediatrics & Child Health*, *14*(5), 315–318.

Lam, L. T. (2014). Mental health literacy and mental health status in adolescents: A population-based survey. *Child and Adolescent Psychiatry and Mental Health*, *8*(1), 26–34.

Larson, R. W., Rickman, A. N., Gibbons, C. M. & Walker, K. C. (2009). Practitioner expertise: Creating quality within the daily tumble of events in youth settings. *New Directions for Youth Development*, *2009*(121), 71–88.

LivingWorks Education. (2007). *Applied suicide intervention skills training: Trainer's manual* (X.1.5 ed.). Calgary, AB: Author.

Mancuso, J. M. (2008). Health literacy: A concept/dimensional analysis. *Nursing and Health Sciences*, *10*, 248–255.

Mayo, P. (2004). *Liberating praxis: Paulo Freire's legacy for radical education and politics*. Westport, CT: Praeger.

Mazzer, K. R., Rickwood, D. J. & Vanags, T. (2012). Teachers and sports coaches supporting people's mental health: Promotion, prevention and early intervention. *World Academy of Science, Engineering and Technology*, *66*, 489–494.

McDaniel, C. (2004). Critical literacy: A questioning stance and the possibility for change. *The Reading Teacher*, *57*(5), 472–481.

Menezes de Souza, L. M. T. (2007). Editor's preface. *Critical Literacy: Theories and Practices*, *1*(1), 4–5. Retrieved from http://www. criticalliteracyjournal.org/ cljournalissue1volume1.pdf

Merton, B. (2004). *An evaluation of the impact of youth work in England* (Research Report RR606, Department of Education & Skills). Nottingham, England: De Montfort

Expertise. Retrieved from http://webarchive.nationalarchives.gov.uk/ 20130401151715/ http://www.education.gov.uk/publications/eOrderingDownload/RR606.pdf

New London Group. (2000). A pedagogy of multiliteracies: Designing social futures. In B. Cope & M. Kalantzis (Eds.), *Multiliteracies: Literacy learning and the design of social futures* (pp. 9–37). New York, NY: Routledge.

Norton, B. (2007). Critical literacy and international development. *Critical literacy: Theories and practices*, *1*(1), 6–15.

Olsson, D. P. & Kennedy, M. G. (2010). Mental health literacy among young people in a small US town: Recognition of disorders and hypothetical helping responses. *Early Intervention in Psychiatry*, *4*(4), 291–298.

Pelkonen, M. & Marttunen, M. (2003). Child and adolescent suicide: Epidemiology, risk factors, and approaches to prevention. *Pediatric Drugs*, *5*(4), 243–263.

Prinsloo, M. & Baynham, M. (2008). Introduction: Renewing literacy studies. In M. Prinsloo & M. Baynham (Eds.), *Literacies, global and local* (pp. 1–13). Philadelphia, PA: John Benjamins.

Purcell, R., Goldstone, S., Moran, J., Albiston, D., Edwards, J., Pennell, K. & McGorry, P. (2011). Toward a twenty-first century approach to youth mental health care: Some Australian initiatives. *International Journal of Mental Health*, *40*(2), 72–87.

Ranahan, P. (2013a). Being with: Child and youth care professionals' practice with suicidal adolescents. *Relational Child and Youth Care Practice*, *26*(1), 6–17.

Ranahan, P. (2013b). Pathways for preparation: Locating suicide education in preparing professionals for encounters with suicidal adolescents. *Child & Youth Services*, *34*(4), 387–401.

Ranahan, P. (2013c). "Why did you call for them?" Child and youth care professionals' practice of flooding the zone during encounters with suicidal adolescents. *Child Care in Practice*, *19*(2), 138–161.

Ranahan, P. (2014). Watching in child and youth care suicide interventions: The potential for observation practices to be disengaging. *International Journal of Child, Youth and Family Studies*, *5*(1), 4–23.

Ranahan, P. & Pellissier, R. (2015). Being green: A discourse analysis of youth workers' talk of initial touchstone experiences with suicidal youth. *Relational Child and Youth Care Practice*, *27*(4), 11-22.

Rickwood, D., Deane, F. P., Wilson, C. (2007). When and how do young people seek professional help for mental health problems? *The Medical Journal of Australia*, *187*(Suppl. 7), S35–S39.

Rootman, I., Frankish, J. & Kaszap, M. (2007). Health literacy: A new frontier. In M. O'Neill, S. Dupéré, A. Pederson, & I. Rootman (Eds.), *Health promotion in Canada: Critical perspectives* (2nd ed., pp. 61–74). Toronto, ON: Canadian Scholars' Press.

Scribner, S. (1984). Literacy in three metaphors. *American Journal of Education*, *93*(1), 6–21.

Shaw, D., Fernandes, J. R. & Rao, C. (2005). Suicide in children and adolescents: A 10-year retrospective review. *American Journal of Forensic Medicine and Pathology*, *26*(4), 309–315.

Sheffield, J. K., Fiorenza, E. & Sofronoff, K. (2004). Adolescents' willingness to seek psychological help: Promoting and preventing factors. *Journal of Youth and Adolescence*, *33*(6), 495–507.

Shor, I. (1999). What is critical literacy? *Journal for Pedagogy, Pluralism & Practice. 4*(1). Retrieved from http://www.lesley.edu/journal-pedagogy-pluralism-practice/ira-shor/critical-literacy/

Spence, J. (2008). What do you youth workers do? Communicating youth work. *Youth Studies Ireland*, *2*(2), 3–18.

Street, B. V. (1995). *Social literacies: Critical approaches to literacy in development, ethnography and education*. Essex, England: Pearson Education.

Street, B. V. (2009). The future of 'social literacies.' In M. Baynham & M. Prinsloo (Eds.), *The future of literacy studies* (pp. 21–37). New York, NY: Palgrave Macmillan.

Strong-Wilson, T. (2006). Re-visioning one's narratives: Exploring the relationship between researcher self-study and teacher research. *Studying Teacher Education*, *2*(1), 59–76.

Wang, J., Adair, C., Fick, G., Lai, D., Evans, B., Waye Perry, B. … Addington, D. (2007). Depression literacy in Alberta: Findings from a general population sample. *Canadian Journal of Psychiatry*, *52*(7), 442–449.

Wexler, L. M. & Gone, J. P. (2012). Culturally responsive suicide prevention in Indigenous communities: Unexamined assumptions and new possibilities. *American Journal of Public Health*, *102*(5), 800–806.

Wexler, L. M., White, J. & Trainor, B. (2015). Why an alternative to suicide prevention gatekeeper training is needed for rural Indigenous communities: Presenting an empowering community storytelling approach. *Critical Public Health*, *25*(2), 205–217.

White, J. (2012). Youth suicide as a "wild" problem: Implications for prevention practice. *Suicidology Online*, *3*, 42–50.

White, J. & Morris, J. (2010). Precarious spaces: Risk, responsibility and uncertainty in school-based suicide prevention programs. *Social Sciences & Medicine*, *71*(12), 2187–2194.

White, J. & Stoneman, L. (2012). Thinking and doing prevention: A critical analysis of contemporary youth crime and suicide prevention discourses. *Child & Youth Services*, *33*, 104–126.

Wilson, C. J. & Deane, F. P. (2001). Adolescent opinions about reducing help-seeking barriers and increasing appropriate help engagement. *Journal of Educational and Psychological Consultation*, *12*(4), 345–364.

Wood, J. W. (2002, April). *Defining literacies*. Paper presented at the Annual Meeting of Educational Research Association, New Orleans, LA.

In: Adolescent Health Literacy and Learning
Editors: D. L. Begoray and E. M. Banister
ISBN: 978-1-63482-897-0

Chapter 9

Addressing Girls' Health Literacy and Learning with Young Adult 'Problem' Novels

Deborah Begoray[1], **Elizabeth Banister**[2] and **Sabrena Jaswal**[3]*
[1]Department of Curriculum and Instruction, University of Victoria, Canada
[2]School of Nursing, University of Victoria, Canada
[3]Independent Researcher, UK

Abstract

This chapter promotes the usefulness of using young adult problem novels as a way to open discussion with adolescent girls about health and wellness issues. Eleven novels were chosen from a list of award winners as ones that presented a high-quality reading experience for middle and high school adolescents and an accurate portrayal of a health problem, such as bullying, eating disorders, cutting, cancer, death, dating relationships, rape, drug and alcohol abuse. Each novel's health issue is discussed with supporting citations and ways that teachers and health educators might use these novels in classrooms or clinical settings. The authors conclude that not only are problem novels useful for adolescent girls' learning but will also help to educate adults about the modern health concerns of these girls.

Keywords: girls, problem novels, health risks, health literacy

Introduction

Focusing Questions

1. How do you think young adult problem novels might help adolescent readers develop greater understanding of the health problems they and other adolescents may experience?

* Correspondence author (email): dbegoray@uvic.ca.

2. How can problem novels be used to help adolescents develop greater health literacy?

As a group of women and health literacy scholars, we hold the health literacy and health behaviours of adolescent girls (12–19 years of age) as a primary interest. For these girls, disease results primarily from risky health behaviours (Centers for Disease Control and Prevention, 2013). We need effective approaches to reach these girls "where they are" (Begoray & Banister, 2007, p. 24), helping them to learn about their physical and emotional health in a holistic way that acknowledges the complexity of their lives.

Young adult novels — those written for an adolescent audience and "narrated through a young adult consciousness" (Belbin, 2011, p. 141) — are one promising resource to help girls understand health issues both cognitively and emotionally. The use of novels offers opportunities for discussing various interpretations about health concerns and can help with problem solving, interacting imaginatively with those affected, and for adopting suitable behaviours and attitudes toward health issues, including cultural ones (Perkin & Rodriquez, 2013; Pytash, 2013). The use of novels "can increase the number of learning tools available" (Perkin & Rodriquez, 2013, p. 758) for health practitioners and educators. Indeed, literature, books, pamphlets, songs, stories, and so on have been used since ancient times for promoting therapeutic gain that "can foster insight and a deeper understanding of self, help readers find solutions to personal problems, develop life skills, and enhanced self-image" (McCulliss & Chamberlain, 2013, p. 14). Such uses of novels can assist young women to address health issues in their own lives and can provide the adults in their lives — parents, grandparents, health practitioners — to understand them better.

The use of young adult literature combined with reader response (Rosenblatt, 1978) activities is one way health educators can assist adolescents to think critically about novels and about the many adverse health challenges they may confront now or in the future. These health issues include challenges in dating relationships (e.g., sexual assault from dating partner, unplanned pregnancy), peer relationships (e.g., bullying), confronting illness (e.g., cancer), and other behaviours (e.g., disordered eating, alcohol and drug abuse, suicide). In this chapter, we discuss 11 novels that we believe have excellent potential to address health literacy and learning objectives for adolescent girls both in the classroom and in clinics. In addition, we suggest several activities educators and practitioners can use to help these adolescents engage with the health issues raised in these novels.

Choice of Novels

Young adult *problem novels* (i.e., a realistic novel centred on an issue that challenges the main character) or *trauma novels* (Balaev, 2008) were chosen to cover a number of health challenges faced by adolescent girls. The novels were all of high literary quality, almost all were award winners, and were either recommended by teachers and librarians or known personally by one or more of the chapter authors. We then narrowed our selection to novels addressing health issues that adolescent girls identified in our own research on adolescent sexual health and sexual health education (Banister & Begoray, 2006; Banister, Begoray, & Daly, 2011). These novels had an adolescent girl as the main character. We chose mostly works that used first-person narrators because of their intimate voice and potential appeal to adolescent girls. Finally, we chose novels from different countries and cultures, including Canadian Indigenous culture, to provide examples to show readers that adolescent health concerns are shared by girls in other places and other ethnic groups.

ADOLESCENT GIRLS' HEALTH NEEDS

Research indicates that adolescent girls face a number of serious health issues such as unplanned pregnancy, sexually transmitted infections (Centers for Disease Control and Prevention, 2013), smoking (Health Canada, 2014), disordered eating (Stice, Marti, Shaw, & Jaconis, 2009), self-injurious behaviour (Brunner et al., 2014), and substance and alcohol abuse (Flegel, 2013). The prevalence of dating violence among adolescents is also widespread (Niolon et al., 2015; World Health Organization [WHO], 2014). Despite such health challenges, research has shown how health-promoting interventions can enhance adolescents' strengths and improve their perspective on events, which builds hope for the future (Barry, Clarke, Jenkins, & Patel, 2013; Guse et al., 2012). Teachers are one group that can play a significant role in promoting and improving adolescents' health (Cheng & Wong, 2015) and health literacy (Kostenius, 2013). Other adults important in adolescents' health lives are, of course, parents and health practitioners.

Adolescence is a time when young people experiment and engage in new experiences — both positive and negative. Adolescents are usually aware that they are at risk for health problems and want to discuss their concerns with adults they trust (Kadivar et al., 2014). In addition to having opportunities to talk about their health (Alexander et al., 2014), adolescents require accurate health information (Smart, Parker, Lampert, & Sulo, 2012; Vardavas, Kondilis, Patelarou, Akrivos, & Falagas, 2009). In addition, they may be subject to unintended events by virtue of their inexperience, lack of physical strength, or exposure to risky environments. Young adult problem novels featuring health topics provide one avenue for initiating discussion about these issues.

ADOLESCENT GIRLS' HEALTH EDUCATION NEEDS

Transferring knowledge and the teaching of skills is a primary function of most school health education programs yet little evidence exists to show positive influences on adolescent health using current approaches (Jackson, Henderson, Frank, & Haw, 2012). Gone are the days when giving students a textbook and a list of questions to be answered can be defended as effective health education. Dusty brochures in clinics are similarly questionable as able to engage adolescent interest. Rather, teenagers need health educators who are willing to broach health topics in a sensitive, direct, nonjudgmental, and open manner (Elfers et al., 2014). Educators need access to strategies and resources that are proven to be effective in reaching these students (Pytash, 2013). Resources (e.g., reading materials) need to be carefully chosen to address adolescents' need for general information and specific examples. To be effective, any teaching approach needs to reflect a thorough understanding of adolescents' perspectives of their health (Spencer, 2013) and their developmental appropriateness (Zimmerman, 2013).

YOUNG ADULT NOVELS DEPICTING HEALTH PROBLEMS

Young adult novels that describe challenging health experiences candidly and sensitively are particularly helpful bridges to engage teens in thinking about adolescents' lived experiences; such novels often focus on sensitive health issues and provide the opportunity "to gain insight into human nature, explore emotion that may seem puzzling or troubling, and reflect on the consequences without engaging in these acts" (Pytash, 2013, p. 477). Trade books (i.e., books intended for public sale as opposed to books specifically for school settings) have a number of advantages for helping teachers to engage adolescent readers: variety, interest and relevance, and comprehensibility (McGowan & Guzzetti as cited in Vacca, Vacca, & Begoray, 2005).

Variety

Resources for reading in health education classrooms are usually textbooks from which students are expected to learn health facts. Novels offer variety in reading assignments and an expanded perspective that includes emotional content. Contemporary novels "are inherently relevant in that, by design, they are responsive to the emotional and cultural challenges young people face in their everyday lives" (Ivey & Johnston, 2013, p. 257).

Interest and Relevance

Novels are meant primarily to be interesting: "[t]he combination of storytelling and informing is an ancient concept that can be traced to the beginnings of the oral tradition when storytellers were the newscasters, entertainers, and teachers who kept society intact and growing" (Vacca et al., 2005, p. 36). Novels actively engage adolescent readers with a character relating her own story, helping readers to see events as she describes them.

Relevance is also a major feature of the problem novel. Adolescents want to know about the lives of other adolescents who are involved in experiences that seem realistic to them. Research has shown that adolescents need to be engaged by novels if they are to involve themselves in learning. Ivey (2012) discovered that Grade 8 students were "drawn to edgy, sometimes gritty, contemporary young adult fiction" (p. 184) and, furthermore, that they chose novels dealing with issues such as substance abuse and addiction, gang violence and bullying "among other mature topics" (p. 186). The novels' setting mattered less than adolescents' perception that they could identify with the story's characters; that is, a teen in a rural community could become interested in a narrative taking place in a big city.

Comprehensibility

Problem novels can help bridge adolescents to understand more challenging health issues. Adolescent girls, for example, are often called upon to have an advanced understanding of health risk and the physical and emotional consequences of their actions. As these girls mature, they may have to deal with difficult health issues personally or indirectly through the experiences of family or friends. Even if they do not encounter such problems, reading novels with health topics can help them to develop empathy or to recognize that others have feelings that must be taken into account during interactions (Ivey, 2012; Luce-Kapler, Sumara, & Iftody, 2010). Comprehending the personal cost of health issues can be initially taught and normalized with novels that portray events and characters' reactions: "young people can benefit from a range of excellent stories reflecting vastly different characters whose experiences are both familiar and unfamiliar to readers" (Johnson-Copenhaver & Copenhaver, 2007, p. 39). Fortunately, there are a large number of young adult novels that both appeal to adolescent girls and deal with health issues in an honest way.

THE ELEVEN NOVELS

The 11 female protagonists who appear in the novels discussed below range from 14–18 years of age though most are 14 or 15 years old. Students in Grades 8–10 are an appropriate audience for these novels; parents, teachers, or health practitioners may decide to individually recommend them to younger (i.e., ages 12 or 13 years) or older adolescents as appropriate to their health challenges, maturity, and reading ability.

The Beckoners

The Beckoners (Mac, 2004) is set in a Canadian high school. This novel has won a number of awards including the 2005 *White Ravens International Youth Library Selection of Outstanding Books*. The eponymous gang are an incredibly aggressive and violent all-female group. Fifteen-year-old Zoe, who has moved from another town with her mother and infant half-sister, joins the gang but finds it increasingly difficult to reconcile its activities with her own values. When another girl, April, is bullied by gang members who then kill her dog, Zoe becomes determined to put an end to the gang's violent ways:

> Zoe watched the girls watch the police arrive. She'd read somewhere once that serial killers start out by hurting animals. Did they know that? Which one of them actually did it, she wondered. Brady? Beck? Had they been stoned? Drunk? High on the hype of each other? (p. 207)

This book takes a candid look at bullying, its victims and perpetrators, and the problems that can arise when schools and adults turn a blind eye to its presence. "Targeted use of books that deal with bullies and bullying is one way for classroom teachers to address, and perhaps deter, this behavior." (Entenman, Murnen, & Hendricks, 2005, p. 361). The Canadian Association for Public Health (2011) noted the increase in bullying especially amongst girls: 71% of Grade 10 girls now report bullying ranging from physical harm to social exclusion and online shaming. Bullying has long-lasting impacts on future health behaviours as well. Adults may want to pair this novel with other anti-bullying resources available online such as the video *To This Day* by Vancouver spoken-word artist Shane Koyczan (2013).

Cut

Cut (McCormick, 2000) is an American novel that tells the story of Callie, a 15-year-old girl in a treatment facility for cutting herself. For Callie, cutting is a coping mechanism. She remains almost totally mute (see this silencing phenomenon also in *Speak* described below) through the majority of this story as she attends both group and individual therapy. Eventually Callie starts to speak to those around her. As the story progresses, readers realize why she began cutting herself and the role that her dysfunctional family had in her self-mutilation. An early scene describes Callie's first experience cutting herself:

> a perfect, straight line of blood bloomed from under the edge of the blade. The line grew into a long, fat bubble, a lush crimson bubble that got bigger and bigger. I watched from above, waiting to see how big it would get before it burst. When it did, I felt awesome. Satisfied, finally. (p. 3)

The imagery is vivid and compelling, engaging for adolescent readers. It portrays an emotion that can help adolescent girls' better understand the experiences and health challenges of the main character. It can also provide parents and other adults with insight into cutting behaviours. Educators may want to pair this novel with *Wintergirls*, discussed below, that also deals with cutting.

Go Ask Alice

Go Ask Alice (Anonymous, 1971) is the diary of a troubled 15-year-old girl growing up in a middle-class American household in the 1960s. While controversy about the real or fictional nature of the diary exists, the girl, who is never identified by name, struggles with a number of issues that still resonate with adolescent girls today. The main character feels alone and believes that she does not fit in at school or at home. She suffers from a number of insecurities including a poor body image:

> I've lost ten pounds. I'm down to a hundred and fifteen pounds which is all right, but I'd still like to lose another ten pounds. Mom says I don't want to get that thin, but she doesn't know! I do! I do! I do! (p. 6)

A chance encounter with drugs at a party leads to a downward spiral of habitual drug use and promiscuity. (A similar drug abuse initiation forms part of the plot in *Crank*, described below.)

Despite the period in which this book is set, the diary entries are timeless. Early in the novel, the girl has her first experience with drug use and writes in her diary: "It was fun! It was ecstatic! It was glorious! But I don't think I'll ever try it again. I've heard too many frightening stories about drugs." (p. 26). However, her resolve crumbles and by late in the book she is sadder and wiser: "Anyone who says pot and acid are not addicting is a damn, stupid, raving idiot, unenlightened fool." She berates herself for her naiveté: "All the time pretending to myself that I could take it or leave it!" (p. 72). The novel's epilogue suggests that the main character dies of an overdose. The topic will resonate with many adolescents given that experimenting with drug and alcohol use is common among this population (Flegel, 2013).

Teachers, health practitioners, or parents might ask adolescents to compare the experiences of 'the girl' with those of Kristina in *Crank*, discussed below. Do they think that the gap of 30 years between publication dates shows that teens have different experiences with drug abuse now than in 1971? They could then write a dialog between these two girls in which they compare their experiences. Students/clients could also be asked to do research online using a site such as MedlinePlus (www.nlm.nih.gov/medlineplus/) to further research the effects of various illicit drugs on adolescents. Opening up conversations with teens about drug abuse is vitally important for parents especially. There are a number of helpful online sites offering further ideas such as Tween and Teen Health that is maintained by the Mayo Clinic (www.mayoclinic.org/healthy-living/tween-and-teen-health/in-depth/teen-drug-abuse/art-20045921).

Crank

Crank (Hopkins, 2004) is an American novel told in a series of poems in the voice of the 16-year-old main character, Kristina Snow. Crank is crystal methamphetamine, which Kristina calls 'the monster.' In a poem, Flirtin' with the Monster, she writes: "Life was good before I met the monster. After, life was great. At least for a little while." (p. 1). Kristina is growing up with her divorced mother, a stepfather, and two siblings. She leaves to spend the summer with her father in Nevada. She discovers that he is not interested in her but rather in pursuing his interests in women and drugs. Her life goes rapidly downhill when she is introduced to crystal meth at a party by a boy she thinks is a new friend. Kristina returns home to her mother's house but is consumed by the need for crank. She learns to lie and steal and finally is raped in her quest for money to feed her habit. As the book ends, she is 17 and has a baby boy. Kristina still hears the siren song of the monster and continues to use crystal meth.

Crystal meth is known to be highly addictive, leading not only to short-term energy, euphoria, and increased libido but also to paranoia, depression, and fatal seizures (Alberta Health Services, 2010). It has recently been reported that use of crystal meth has spiked 45% in the province of Alberta due to falling prices and easy availability (Canadian Broadcasting Company, 2013). This book is a powerful cautionary tale on a variety of health-related topics — not least the importance of parents as models of behaviour and as guides for adolescent girls with questions on substance use.

Readers of *Crank* will be interested to know that the story is loosely based on the addiction of the author's daughter; it was the first in a trilogy followed by *Glass* (Hopkins, 2007) and *Fallout* (Hopkins, 2014) that continue Kristina's story. Girls may be interested in discussing *Crank* and *Go Ask Alice* together.

Massive

Massive (Bell, 2002) is set in England and examines the struggle that 14-year-old Carmen, her mother, and her grandmother have with food. Carmen, like her grandmother, starts off as an overeater, in stark contrast with her mother who starves herself and is obsessed with exercising and dieting. Following family upheaval involving an abrupt move to another town and her mother's incessant comments about being thin, Carmen becomes bulimic. The story illustrates the plight of individuals suffering from eating disorders and the impact it has on family and friends.

"Media effectively transmits and reinforces certain sociocultural messages, including a thin-ideal body image for girls" (Benowitz-Fredericks, Garcia, Massey, Vasagar, & Borzekowski, 2012, p. 698), which often include dieting products and messages. In this novel, for example, Carmen and her grandmother sit and watch *Inch Loss Island*, a fictional weight-loss television reality show:

> The presenter's lip gloss shimmers as she tells how Wendy got fat when she was pregnant and how she's come to the island to get her figure back. 'It's probably water retention,' she advises. 'I expect the pounds will drop off next week.' (Bell, 2002, p. 37)

Carmen is aware of how false this opinion is but believes as well that she cannot cope with her life without either under- or overeating. The media-manipulated false reality of television and its depictions of food and eating in this novel can provide an opening for conversations with adolescents about nutrition and body image.

The Canadian Association for Public Health (2011) reported that 40% of adolescent girls considered themselves to be "too fat ... [h]owever, only 15% of those Grade 10 adolescent girls were actually overweight or obese based on their self-reported heights and weights" (n.p.). The American Psychological Association (APA; 2015) noted, "As adolescent girls attempt to reconcile the reality of their bodies with the unrealistic and unattainable cultural demands for female thinness, large numbers of girls experience intense body image dissatisfaction" (§ Body image, para. 1). Providing and discussing problem novels such as *Massive* might help in "promot[ing] acceptance of a broad range of appearances, provid[ing] support for individuality and healthy development and play[ing] an instrumental role in protecting adolescent girls from the development of eating and weight-related concerns." (§ Body image, para. 3). Educators may want to pair this novel with *The Earth, My Butt, and Other Big Round Things*, described below.

Speak

Speak (Anderson, 1999), an American novel, was the winner of the 2000 *Michael L. Printz Award for Excellence in Young Adult Literature Honor Book*. Grade 9 student Melinda Sordino lives in a household where communication is primarily done via sticky notes. As the novel begins, her school life is even more silent as her former friends no longer speak to her. She is known at school as the girl who called the police at a summer party involving underage drinking. What she has not disclosed to anyone is that she was raped at that party by an older boy. Melinda suffers in silence as she begins junior high school. Her grades slip, she skips classes, and she has trouble speaking up for herself. She also exhibits other troubling behaviours such as ignoring her physical hygiene and nervously biting her lip. These signs of trauma all largely go unquestioned by the adults in her life except, finally, for an observant teacher. Research tells us that an empathic teacher is often the first to hear girls' direct accounts about difficult life events (Cohall et al., 2007). Supportive relationships with an adult can contribute to positive youth development and reduce adolescents' risky behaviour (Wang, Brinkworth, & Eccles, 2013). As in *The Earth, My Butt and Other Big Round Things*, described below, art activities allow the main character to regain her voice.

Novels such as *Speak* excel in portraying the emotional dimension of sexual assault and may well be termed *trauma literature*: "works of fiction that convey ... profound loss or intense fear" (Balaev, 2008, p. 150). This book vividly describes disturbing experiences. Near the end of the novel, Melinda is once again trapped with her attacker:

> His mouth is on my face. I twist my head. His lips are wet; his teeth knock against my cheekbone. I pull my arms again and he slams his body against mine. I have no legs. My heart wobbles. His teeth are on my neck. The only sound I can make is a whimper. (Anderson, 1999, p. 194)

While we hope that none of our students will ever face a sexual assault, such hopes are naive given the prevalence of the problem. The APA (2015) reported that dating violence is experienced by 10% of high school girls and 22% of university aged women — numbers that might be low given the reluctance of many young women to report incidents. Novels such as *Speak* may lead students to look at wider acts of violence against girls. In 2014, the WHO announced that:

> In recognition of the importance of investing in and empowering girls during adolescence and preventing and eliminating the various forms of violence they experience, the theme of International Day of the Girl Child for 2014 is 'Empowering Adolescent Girls: Ending the Cycle of Violence.' (para. 1)

Educators and parents may also encourage girls to inquire into worldwide violence against girls and women.

The Earth, My Butt and Other Big Round Things

In *The Earth, My Butt and Other Big Round Things* (Mackler, 2003), 15-year-old Virginia feels like an outsider at school and even in her own family. When her best and only friend leaves New York City for Walla Walla, Washington, Virginia finds herself alone with her problems. She struggles to establish a first relationship with a boy, to lose weight, and to find herself. This novel was a 2004 *Michael L. Printz Honor Book for Excellence in Young Adult Literature*.

As in *Massive,* the lead character has a thin mother who eats salad and exercises obsessively. She offers Virginia advice on dressing in layers and in colours such as beige to cover up her body. It has been established that "[i]n girls, a drive for thinness, or the willingness to alter one's body to meet the social ideal of physical attractiveness, was correlated with parental encouragement to lose weight and the mothers' dieting behaviors" (Benowitz-Fredericks et al., 2012, p. 696). But Virginia breaks out of her life of crash dieting and self-imposed isolation and begins to dress herself in tight purple outfits with matching hair and eye makeup. She gets an eyebrow ring and finds a group of friends including a boyfriend. Together, they work to establish an online magazine or webzine:

> After everyone's introduced themselves, I talk a little about my vision for the webzine. I make sure to add that it will reflect what's going on in all of our heads. Basically, I want it to voice the things that people don't ordinarily talk about. (Mackler, 2003, p. 230)

Virginia also starts to stand up to her parents. When her father tells her he thinks she is slimming down, she replies: "'Dad, we're trying to be more open with each other, right?' Dad nodded, but his forehead wrinkled in confusion. 'Then I have to tell you I'd rather you didn't talk about my body. It's just not yours to discuss.'" (p. 235).

Body image is perhaps one of the major issues faced by adolescent girls. As they reach puberty, they add fat and their hips broaden, taking them further away from societal ideals of thinness (Benowitz-Fredericks et al., 2012), while boys add muscle, which brings them closer to the ideal body for men. Girls who find themselves negatively compared to media images of women may find novels such as *The Earth, My Butt and Other Big Round Things* and *Massive* reassuring. Educators can involve girls in activities that Virginia undertakes such as getting involved in photography and online publishing. Zines are "underground publications that are self-authored and self-edited to allow those who are often unheard to be recognized. Through zining, young women take up topics of importance to them" (Guzzetti, 2012, p. 54). Health educators and parents might encourage girls to join online communities that read and create zines through websites such as GURL (www.gurl.com).

Please Ignore Vera Dietz

As the American novel *Please Ignore Vera Dietz* (King, 2010) begins, Vera is 18 years old and trying to be invisible. She has an absent mother, a distracted father, and a dead boyfriend. Vera works delivering pizzas while trying to keep up at school and to understand her confused thoughts and emotions surrounding her long-standing relationship with Charlie, who recently died. Charlie had had problems of his own: an abusive father, an emotionally absent and abused mother, a manipulative other girlfriend, drug and alcohol abuse. Charlie made a lot of decisions that dismayed Vera and eventually cost him his life. She attempts to unravel the mystery of his final days, create a better relationship with her father, and deal with her own risky behaviours. This novel was a 2011 *Michael L. Printz Honor Book for Excellence in Young Adult Literature*.

Vera is haunted by Charlie especially when she drinks to excess. During what she calls her first real date after his death, she drinks and finds herself in a risky sexual situation. But when she briefly opens her eyes, all she sees are 'Charlies': "They are in the car—all thousand of them, stacked like paper ... pressed against my back, my sides, staring at me. Today they're wearing Charlies' favorite blue and white checked flannel shirt ... I struggle to breathe and can't inhale at all" (p. 116). She knows she owes it to Charlie to clear his name but feels betrayed by him. Teachers and health practitioners may want to focus especially on Vera's need to work through her confusion and learn to cope without using alcohol.

As in *Crank* and *The Earth, My Butt and Other Big Round Things*, a lack of appropriate parental support has a major bearing on Vera's problems. The Canadian Centre for Substance Abuse (2014) advised that almost a third of Canadian teens binge drink; that is, they consume five or more drinks at one time. Adolescents need help from parents, teachers, and health practitioners in understanding that:

> [d]rinking alcohol can lead youth to make bad decisions, such as driving after drinking or getting into a car with a driver who has been drinking. Drinking is also related to increased chances of suicide, homicide, drowning and experiencing or committing physical or sexual assault because alcohol impairs judgment, reasoning and the ability to evaluate risk. (p. 2)

Parents have a major role to play in the health of their children, not just in childhood but in adolescence as well (Community Preventive Services Task Force, 2012; Galloway, 2010). Parents and educators can engage adolescent girls in incorporating school-based drug prevention programs for mitigating the early initiation of alcohol consumption and address risk factors such as peer pressure.

Tilly: A Story of Hope and Resilience

Tilly: A Story of Hope and Resilience (Gray Smith, 2013) centres on a young Indigenous woman in Canada. It is set in the 1980s and is loosely based on the life experiences of the author. The story begins with young Tilly encountering racism for the first time when an angry man on the street refers to her mother as a "Goddamn squaw" (p. 16). Tilly had known she was Lakota on her father's side; after the incident, she realizes her mother is Aboriginal and that she is of mixed ancestry of Scottish, Lakota, and Cree. Tilly grew up learning traditional teachings from her beloved paternal grandmother, who taught her to "be proud of who you are … proud to be an Indian" (p. 25). When her grandmother dies unexpectedly, Tilly's anchor is ripped from her. She slips into a destructive path of alcoholism after a Grade 7 classmate offers her an alcoholic beverage during school lunch break; Tilly accepts the drink to break her loneliness and fit in with peers. Eventually hitting rock bottom, she realizes she needs to change. With the help of mentors, such as her Grade 10 teacher and a Native friendship counselor (an Ojibway woman), she embarks on a courageous journey of finding herself and learning about her ancestors and the teachings they left behind.

The novel brings to the forefront the 20th century history of Indigenous people in Canada, including forced cultural displacement, residential schools, and tuberculosis hospitals. The story illustrates the negative effects of racism on Indigenous youth (Priest, Paradies, Stewart, & Luke, 2011) and the importance of connecting Indigenous youth with traditional teachings and their cultural heritage and resilience for enhancing their mental health (Markstrom, 2011; West, Williams, Suzukovich, Strangeman, & Novins, 2012).

"Adolescents exist within and navigate a racialized society… discussions of race and racism are often marginalized and muted" (Park, 2012, p. 635). Teachers and health educators can facilitate critical conversations with young adult literature to "critique systems of oppression and to empower students" (Schieble, 2012, p. 212); such critique needs to attend to both "the reading context and sociopolitical histories and identities involving the reader and text" (p. 213). Teachers can use the novel to engage students in reading and writing to make visible a variety of institutional privileges that benefit whites and generally go unnoticed (Schieble, 2012). For example, in Canada Aboriginal youth continue to carry an increased burden of illness and to be disadvantaged in comparison to non-Aboriginals. There are still socioeconomic deprivations and inequalities within the Canadian education and health care system (Kaspar, 2013). Using a lens of whiteness acknowledges how "white-dominated institutions such as schools committed grave injustices in the forced assimilation and language policies that stripped Indigenous peoples of their cultural identities and practices" (Schieble, 2012, p. 216). *Tilly* received the 2014 *Burt Award for First Nations, Métis and Inuit Literature First Prize*. As with *Please Ignore Vera Dietz*, this book can offer readers insight into the disempowering effects of alcohol misuse for all adolescent girls — Aboriginal and non-Aboriginal — and help them consider how to handle risky situations and potential outcomes resulting from excessive alcohol use.

Wintergirls

Wintergirls (Anderson, 2009), an American novel, focuses on 18-year-old Lia who is suffering from anorexia and how she deals with her friend's death from the same disorder. The novel provides graphic details of Lia's spiral into intense guilt and self-harming behaviour after learning that Cassie died alone in a motel room. Lia and Cassie were *wintergirls* competing to be the thinnest; prior to her death, Cassie leaves Lia a voicemail message that tells Lia she won the contest. The reader is privy to Lia's internal conflict, illustrating a nightmare of self-hatred: "stupid/ugly/bitch/fat/stupid/baby/stupid/loser/stupid/lost" (p. 60).

Tension builds as Lia struggles to save her own life. The novel weaves in the role of self-forgiveness in recovery. Lia gradually lets down her wall of denial about her illness with a psychiatrist and recognizes her need for medical assistance. She is readmitted to an eating disorder clinic: "Somehow I dragged myself out of the dark and asked for help" (p. 277). The book concludes with a realistic theme of hope: "There is no magic cure, no making it all go away forever. There are only small steps upward; an easier day, an unexpected laugh, a mirror that doesn't matter anymore. I am thawing." (p. 277).

This book illustrates the suffering and isolation of adolescents living with an eating disorder. Graphic details of Lia's emotional and physical deterioration, including self-cutting behavior, confront the reader with the intense pressure for adolescents to meet societal beauty standards of thinness. Adolescent females are significantly more likely than males to develop eating disorders and adolescence is a time of heightened risk (Suisman et al., 2012). Discussions among peers about attaining thinness is one factor that can reinforce and perpetuate thinness among adolescent girls (Suisman et al., 2012). The novel demonstrates the importance of using peer-based strategies that "challenge internalization of the thin ideal" (Keel & Forney, 2013, p. 433). Teachers and health educators can provide opportunities for peer discussion and critique through reading groups or literature circles, perhaps including *Massive* and *The Earth, My Butt and Other Big Round Things,* and offer students opportunities to question each other about why and how they view characters such as Lia in that way (Park, 2012).

The use of visualization as a critical literacy technique can also be used to "support students to become more wide awake about people, both literary and real" (Park, 2012, p. 637). Teachers can invite students to visualize parts of the book (e.g., the character of Lia or her behaviour) that interests or challenges them to help them think about anorexia as a "real issue" (p. 638). As with *Cut*, the vivid imagery of Lia's cutting and emaciation conveys painful emotion that can help adolescents to have empathy for the character's lived experience.

The Fault in Our Stars

The Fault in Our Stars (Green, 2012) won the 2013 *Children's Choice Book Award for Best Teen Book* and was made into a movie with the same title that was released in 2014. The focal character in this American novel is 17-year-old Hannah who has terminal cancer. Although her condition has temporarily stopped deteriorating, as the novel opens she is depressed. She knows she will never be better. Her concerned parents urge her to join a group for teens with cancer where she meets Augustus and gradually falls in love. Hannah and Augustus set out to live their lives together with the knowledge that their relationship will be brief but can also be amazing. When they first kiss, she observes:

> The space around us evaporated, and for a weird moment I really liked my body; this cancer-ruined thing I'd spent years dragging around suddenly seemed worth the struggle, worth the test tubes and the PICC lines and the ceaseless bodily betrayal of the tumors. (p. 203)

But Augustus, too, is living with cancer; together, they face the inevitable.

"About 70,000 adolescents and young adults (ages 15–39 years) are diagnosed with cancer each year in the United States" (National Cancer Institute, n.d., para. 1), and "[e]ach year, on average 412 adolescents are diagnosed with cancer in Canada and 74 die from the disease" (Public Health Agency of Canada, 2012, n.p.). Novels that present the emotional experience of patients with terminal illness without flinching are especially valuable for discussion with adolescents and for the insight of adults who are involved with young adults' health care.

Summary

It is important to note that most young adult problem novels have hopeful endings where characters find their way through the problem, often through discovering inner strengths such as the courage to reach out to others who can help them. In *The Beckoners* for example, Zoe finds that she has friends who are not in the gang with whom she can talk about her problems; these friends then find a way to deal with the gang. Similarly in *Speak*, Melinda finds her voice when another girl points out that graffiti written by many girls on the washroom walls identifies her attacker on a list as "Guys to Stay Away From" (Anderson, 1999, p. 185). Once she is no longer isolated, Melinda can begin to cope with her experience of sexual assault; she says, "I feel like I can fly" (p. 186). In comparison, the two novels on drug use, *Go Ask Alice* and *Crank*, have darker endings, with Alice committing suicide and Kristina leaving her baby with her mother and going to find her next hit of crank.

RESPONSE ACTIVITIES TO BUILD HEALTH KNOWLEDGE

Reader response theory (Rosenblatt, 1978) and research on student engagement (e.g., Ivey, 2012) suggests that adolescents can create their own meaning by combining their own experiences with the ones they encounter in the novel. Health educators can foster such engagement by inviting students to respond to novels. Response assignments are particularly important to foster understanding of the health issues in young adult problem novels such as those described above. Responding to young adult problem novels can be encouraged in a variety of media: writing, visually representing (e.g., drawing, creating videos), and talking.

WRITING/VISUALLY REPRESENTING

Response Journals

Journals in which students write and sketch are a powerful way to get them to think about their personal reactions — thoughts and feelings — in response to a reading. However, pen-and-paper journals are less appealing to adolescents now than online equivalents, such as blogs that support photos and other visuals as well as written text. Boniel-Nissim and Barak (2013), for example, reported that teens who wrote and posted blogs about social and emotional experiences on sites open to response benefited from the experience.

Health literacy skills include accessing information, comprehending and evaluating it, and communicating it to others. Health educators might, therefore, ask adolescents after each book chapter to answer a choice of open-ended questions, such as: What events in this chapter remind you of events in your own life? In other books or stories? In television or movies? What health information do you think the author wants to suggest is healthy or risky? Do you agree? Why or why not? How might you evaluate this information? What other sources of information might you consult? What character or characters would you like to meet? What questions might you ask him/her? If you were the author, what events might you describe in the next chapter? What visual image is the clearest in this chapter? Choose a quotation and/or draw the image.

Health educators assigning response journals, blogs, or threaded discussion groups will have to be prepared to respond to students who may reveal troubling personal events and feelings (Pytash, 2013) by having appropriate supports in place ahead of time (e.g., access to a youth worker or school counsellor). Health practitioners and parents might also suggest that individual girls join online discussion groups or teen book clubs to write about their novels such as those available through a public library or websites such as Goodreads (http://www.goodreads.com/).

Memory Boxes

Adolescents can create a character's diary and keepsakes, then find or create a memory box in which to place them. For example, April in *The Beckoners* might have a diary tracing her bullying, ending with the day when the gang is tricked into confessing their abusive activities. One of her keepsakes might be a picture of her dog Shadow. Memory boxes can serve as beginning points for further activities, for example, writing a dialogue between April and a school counselor where she explains the significance of her keepsakes, or a conversation between April and Zoe 20 years later when they meet at a school reunion and discover that they have each kept their boxes. Photos and videos might be produced and then assembled, creating a character's Facebook™, Instagram™, or Flickr™ pages and engaging adolescent interest in technology and social media.

TALKING

Hot Seat

Adolescents can assume the roles of characters in the novel. Educators will need to make careful choices of which students will be able to play the roles of vulnerable characters. In a classroom or other group setting, it is best to ask students in private and in advance if they would be willing to participate. Staying in character, role-playing students sit facing the class then begin by making a 1-minute comment on their behaviour in the chapter or section of the book. Adolescents playing characters must be prepared to answer questions from other class members based on the novel's events and on related health information that they have sought from other sources. Guiding questions might include: What action are you the most/least proud of in this chapter? Why? How did you feel? How is this behaviour/action healthy or unhealthy? Why are you engaging in it? Then the class can ask the characters questions to which they must answer in character. For example in *Crank,* Kristina might be asked why she didn't just stop taking meth, who she asked for help, and so on. Roleplays can be videotaped and reviewed by students to improve their understanding. Health practitioners might roleplay with individual girls, themselves taking on the role of a difficult character such as a drug-pushing boyfriend so that the girls can practice their responses in the role of the novel's main character.

Think/Pair/Share

Adolescents sometimes need encouragement to think as individuals before sharing with peers. They are generally so sociable, however, that they are eager to hear their classmates' reactions. Think/Pair/Share provides time for personal thought and sharing with others. During the Think stage, adolescents are asked to consider their own answer to an opinion question. For example in the novel *Massive*, students might be asked to write for 2 minutes in response to the task: "Agree or disagree with this statement: Carmen should just eat a healthy diet and ignore her mother and grandmother." After the time allotment, they join in pairs to share their answers and hear from their partner in a further 2-minute conversation. They might then come to an agreed-upon decision. These decisions could be based on further reading from a textbook, Internet sites, or other informational sources. Group decisions could be further shared through the creation of videos and websites for the benefit of other girls.

CONCLUSION

The topics and plot events of young adult problem novels are frequently harrowing and may be difficult for some health educators, especially in schools to consider using in the classroom. For teachers who prefer not to assign such novels, they can be made available in a classroom or school library for students to choose on their own or with teacher or peer recommendation. If teachers elect to take up the challenge, they need to be prepared to defend their use of young adult problem novels with health issues. Teachers need to advise administrators, who are often the first to hear from concerned parents, about why these novels deserve a place in the curriculum. Parents, too, should be encouraged to read these novels.

The overall skill and comfort level of educators about health challenges of adolescents needs attention if health-promoting interactions are to be promoted (Cohall et al., 2007). Many teachers desire additional resources such as inservice workshops to address these needs (Cohall et al., 2007), and these should be provided. Students should be informed about the health-related topics to be covered in the novels, given that some of these topics may be *too close for comfort* and may even re-traumatize adolescents who had experienced a difficult situation. In such instances, students should be offered the choice to either read an alternate, less emotionally evocative work or remove themselves from class discussion. Instances when students do become distraught need to be handled in a sensitive and caring manner. Referral to a mental health professional (e.g., school mental health nurse or counsellor) may be needed (Cooper, Clements, & Holt, 2012). Beginning teachers especially should consult an experienced teacher or their principal for guidance on the choice of young adult problem novels and an approach to engaging adolescents in difficult topics (Pytash, 2013).

Health practitioners who decide to use novels with their patients may face challenges of a different sort: defending the use of fiction in a real health setting. Scholars such as Freeman and Bays (2007) recommend the introduction of nursing students, for example, to the use of novels to increase understanding of adolescents in their future practice. As well, Simon (2014) reminds us: "Experiencing disease, violence, issues of race and sexuality, bereavement, and mental illness on the printed page can help prepare clinicians for clinical encounters with these problems, among others" (p. 356). We suggest that health practitioners who *read* fiction might become those who *use* fiction in their practices with their patients.

These novels and others like them will be popular choices at home, in classrooms, and in waiting rooms. They provide variety, interest and relevance, and comprehensibility; as novels, they provide specific examples of adolescent girls trying to cope with difficult life events, with all the attendant trials and tribulations, but often with success.

NOTE

This chapter has been updated and expanded from an earlier version by Begoray, Banister, and Jaswal (2008).

Questions for Discussion, Reflection, and Writing

1. What are some of your reactions to the health issues described in the novels? What might be some of the challenges for teachers to use problem novels in the classroom?
2. How can educators provide opportunities for adolescents to express their understandings of the novels? How can conversations among peers about the novels be facilitated?
3. How can educators be aware of sensitive issues many adolescents face and engage them in critical thinking about these issues?

List of Online Resources

- The Michael L. Printz Award for Excellence in Young Adult Literature – http://www.ala.org/yalsa/printz
- Canadian Library Association Young Adult Book Award – http://www.cla.ca/AM/Template.cfm?Section=Young_Adult_Canadian_Book_Award&Template=/CM/ContentDisplay.cfm&ContentID=2504
- Johns Hopkins Bloomberg School of Public Health: Center for Adolescent Health – http://www.jhsph.edu/research/centers-and-institutes/center-for-adolescent-health/

REFERENCES

Alberta Health Services. (2010). *Crystal methamphetamine* (Teacher Information Series). Edmonton, AB: Author. Retrieved from http://www.albertahealthservices.ca/AddictionsSubstanceAbuse/if-tch-teacher-info-series-crystal-meth.pdf

Alexander, S. C., Fortenberry, J. D., Pollak, K. I., Bravender, T., Davis, J. K., Østbye, T. ... Shields, C. G. (2014). Sexuality talk during adolescent health maintenance visits. *JAMA Pediatrics*, *168*(2), 163–169.

American Psychological Association. (2015). *A new look at adolescent girls*. Washington, DC: Author. Retrieved from http://www.apa.org/pi/families/ resources/adolescent-girls.aspx

Anderson, L. H. (1999). *Speak*. New York, NY: Penguin Random House.

Anderson, L. H. (2009). *Wintergirls*. New York, NY: Penguin Random House.

Anonymous. (1971). *Go ask Alice*. Englewood Cliffs, NJ: Prentice-Hall.

Balaev, M. (2008). Trends in literary trauma theory. *Mosaic*, *41*(2), 149–165.

Banister, E. & Begoray, D. (2006). A community of practice approach for Aboriginal girls' sexual health education. *Journal of the Canadian Academy of Child and Adolescent Psychiatry*, *15*(4), 168–173.

Banister, E., Begoray, D.. & Daly, L. (2011). Responding to adolescent women's reproductive health concerns: Empowering clients through health literacy. *Health Care for Women International*, *32*(4), 344–354. doi:10.1080/07399332.2010.536603

Barry, M. M., Clarke, A. M., Jenkins, R. & Patel, V. (2013). A systematic review of the effectiveness of mental health promotion interventions for young people in low and middle income countries. *BMC Public Health*, *13*(1), 835. doi:10.1186/1471-2458-13-835

Begoray, D. & Banister, E. (2007). Reaching teenagers where they are: Best practices for girls' sexual health education. *Women's Health & Urban Life Journal*, *4*(1), 24–40.

Begoray, D., Banister, E. & Jaswal, S. (2008). Bridging the gap: Enhancing girls' health literacy through young adult 'problem' novels. *Dragon Lode*, *27*(1), 43–50.

Belbin, D. (2011). What is young adult fiction? *English in Education*, *45*(2), 132–145.

Bell, J. (2002). *Massive*. London, England: Young Picador.

Benowitz-Fredericks, C., Garcia, K., Massey, M., Vasagar, B. & Borzekowski, D. (2012). Body image, eating disorders, and the relationship to adolescent media use. *Pediatric Clinics of North America*, *59*, 693–704.

Boniel-Nissim, M. & Barak, A. (2013). The therapeutic value of adolescents' blogging about social–emotional difficulties. *Psychological Services*, *10*(3), 333–341.

Brunner, R., Kaess, M., Parzer, P., Fischer, G., Carli, V., Hoven, C. W. ... Wasserman, D. (2014). Life-time prevalence and psychosocial correlates of adolescent direct self-injurious behavior: A comparative study of findings in 11 European countries. *Journal of Child Psychology and Psychiatry*, *55*(4), 337–348.

Canadian Association for Public Health. (2011). The health and well-being of Canadian youth and young adults. In D. Butler-Jones, *Chief Public Health Officer's report on the state of public health in Canada, 2011: Youth and young adults – life in transition* (chapter 3). Ottawa, ON: Author. Retrieved from http://www.phac-aspc.gc.ca/cphorsphc-respcacsp/2011/ cphorsphc-respcacsp-06-eng.ph

Canadian Broadcasting Company. (2013). *Crystal meth use on the rise, say Edmonton youth workers*. Toronto, ON: Author. Retrieved from http://www.cbc.ca/news/canada/edmonton/crystal-meth-use-on-the-rise-say-edmonton-youth-workers-1.2419569

Canadian Centre on Substance Abuse. (2014). *Youth and alcohol*. Ottawa, ON: Author. Retrieved from http://www.ccsa.ca/Resource%20Library/CCSA-Youth-and-Alcohol-Summary-2014-en.pdf

Centers for Disease Control and Prevention. (2013). *Youth risk behavior surveillance system (YRBSS)*. Atlanta, GA: Author. Retrieved from http://www.cdc.gov/HealthyYouth/yrbs/index.htm

Cheng, N. Y. I. & Wong, M. Y. E. (2015). Knowledge and attitude of school teachers towards promoting healthy lifestyle to students. *Health*, *7*, 119–126.

Cohall, A. T., Cohall, R., Dye, B., Dini, S., Vaughan R. D. & Coots, S. (2007). Overheard in the halls: What adolescents are saying, and what teachers are hearing, about health issues. *Journal of School Health*, *77*(7), 344–350.

Community Preventive Services Task Force. (2012). Improving adolescent health through interventions targeted to parents and other caregivers: A recommendation. *American Journal of Preventive Medicine*, *42*(3), 327–328.

Cooper, G. D., Clements, P. T. & Holt, K. E. (2012). Examining childhood bullying and adolescent suicide implications for school nurses. *Journal of School Nursing*, *28*(4), 275–283.

Elfers, J., Carlton, L., Gibson, P., Puffer, M., Smith, S. & Todd, K. (2014). The core competencies for adolescent sexual and reproductive health. *American Journal of Sexuality Education*, *9*(1), 81–98.

Entenman, J., Murnen, T. & Hendricks, C. (2005). Victims, bullies and bystanders in K–3 literature: *The Reading Teacher*, *59*(4), 352-364.

Flegel, K. (2013). Big alcohol catches up with girls [Editorial]. *Canadian Medical Association Journal*, *185*(10), 859.

Freeman, L. & Bays, C. (2007). Using literature and the arts to teach nursing. *International Journal of Nursing Education Scholarship*, *4*(1), 1–14.

Galloway, D. (2010). Parents' roles in improving the health of adolescents. *North Carolina Medical Journal*, *71*(4), 383–385.

Gray Smith, M. (2013). *Tilly: A story of hope and resilience*. Winlaw, BC: Sono Nis Press.

Green, J. (2012). *The fault in our stars*. New York, NY: Dutton Books.

Guse, K., Levine, D., Martins, S., Lira, A., Gaarde, J., Westmorland, W. & Gilliam, M. (2012). Interventions using new digital media to improve adolescent sexual health: A systematic review. *Journal of Adolescent Health*, *51*(6), 535–543.

Guzzetti, B. (2012). Girls' zines as a global literacy practice. In B. Guzzetti & T. Bean (Eds.), *Adolescent literacies and the gendered self* (pp. 53–63). New York, NY: Routledge.

Health Canada. (2014). *Summary of results of the youth smoking survey 2012–2013*. Ottawa, ON: Author. Retrieved from http://www.hc-sc.gc.ca/hc-ps/tobac-tabac/research-recherche/stat/_survey-sondage_2012-2013/result-eng.php

Hopkins, E. (2004). *Crank*. New York, NY: McElderry Books.

Hopkins, E. (2007). *Glass*. New York, NY: McElderry Books.

Hopkins, E. (2014). *Fallout*. New York, NY: McElderry Books.

Ivey, G. (2012). "In this little town nothing much ever happens but someday something will": Reading young adult literature from the Blue Ridge foothills. In D. E. Alvermann & K. A. Hinchman (Eds.), *Reconceptualizing the literacies in adolescents' lives: Bridging the everyday/academic divide* (3rd ed., pp. 181–197), New York, NY: Routledge.

Ivey, G. & Johnston, P. H. (2013). Engagement with young adult literature: Outcomes and processes. *Reading Research Quarterly*, *48*(3), 255–275.

Jackson, C. A., Henderson, M., Frank, J. W. & Haw, S. J. (2012). An overview of prevention of multiple risk behaviour in adolescence and young adulthood. *Journal of Public Health*, *34*(Suppl. 1), i31–i40.

Johnson-Copenhaver, J. & Copenhaver, A. R. (2007). Issues of representation in young adult literature with diabetic protagonists. *Dragon Lode*, *25*(2), 39–45.

Kadivar, H., Thompson, L., Wegman, M., Chisholm, T., Khan, M., Eddleton, K. ... Shenkman, E. (2014). Adolescent views on comprehensive health risk assessment and counseling: Assessing gender differences. *Journal of Adolescent Health*, *55*(1), 24–32.

Kaspar, V. (2013). Mental health of Aboriginal children and adolescents in violent school environments: Protective mediators of violence and psychological/nervous disorders. *Social Science & Medicine*, *81*, 70–78.

Keel, P. K. & Forney, K. J. (2013). Psychosocial risk factors for eating disorders. *International Journal of Eating Disorders*, *46*(5), 433–439.

King, A. S. (2010). *Please ignore Vera Dietz.* New York, NY: Random House.

Kostenius, C. (2013). Student-driven health promotion activities. *Health Education*, *113*(5), 407–419.

Koyczan, S. (2013, February 19). *To this day* [Video file]. Retrieved from https://www.youtube.com/watch?v=ltun92DfnPY

Luce-Kapler, R., Sumara, D. & Iftody, T. (2010). Teaching ethical know-how in new literary spaces. *Journal of Adolescent & Adult Literacy*, *53*(7), 536–541.

Mac, C. (2004). *The beckoners*. Victoria, BC: Orca Books.

Mackler, C. (2003). *The earth, my butt and other big round things*. Somerville, MA: Candlewick Press.

Markstrom, C. A. (2011). Identity formation of American Indian adolescents: Local, national, and global considerations. *Journal of Research on Adolescence*, *21*(2), 519–535.

McCormick, P. (2000). *Cut*. New York, NY: Push Scholastic.

McCulliss, D. & Chamberlain, D. (2013). Bibliotherapy for youth and adolescents: School-based application and research. *Journal of Poetry Therapy*, *26*(1), 13–40.

National Cancer Institute. (n.d.) *Adolescents and young adults with cancer*. Bethesda, MD: National Institutes of Health. Retrieved from http://www.cancer.gov/cancertopics/aya

Niolon, P. H., Vivolo-Kantor, A. M., Latzman, N. E., Valle, L. A., Kuoh, H., Burton, T. ... Tharp, A. T. (2015). Prevalence of teen dating violence and co-occurring risk factors among middle school youth in high-risk urban communities. *Journal of Adolescent Health*, *56*(2), S5–S13.

Park, J. Y. (2012). A different kind of reading instruction: Using visualizing to bridge reading comprehension and critical literacy. *Journal of Adolescent & Adult Literacy*, *55*(7), 629–640.

Perkin, J. & Rodriguez, J. (2013). More lit can fit: Using nontraditional literature in dietetics education to enhance cultural competence, cultural literacy, and critical thinking. *Journal of the Academy of Nutrition and Dietetics*, *113*(6), 757–761.

Priest, N., Paradies, Y., Stewart, P. & Luke, J. (2011). Racism and health among urban Aboriginal young people. *BMC Public Health*, *11*(1), 568. doi:10.1186/1471-2458-11-568.

Public Health Agency of Canada. (2012). *Cancer in adolescents in Canada (15–19 years).* Ottawa, ON: Author. Retrieved from http://www.phac-aspc.gc.ca/cd-mc/cancer/fs-fi/cancer-adol/index-eng.php

Pytash, K. E. (2013). Using YA literature to help preservice teachers deal with bullying and suicide. *Journal of Adolescent & Adult Literacy*, *56*(6), 470–479.

Rosenblatt, L. (1978). *The reader, the text, the poem: The transactional theory of the literary work.* Carbondale, IL: Southern Illinois University Press.

Schieble, M. (2012). Critical conversations on whiteness with youth adult literature. *Journal of Adolescent & Adult Literacy*, *56*(3), 212–221.

Simon, H. B. (2014). Reading fiction. *American Journal of Medicine*, *127*(4), 356–357.

Smart, K. A., Parker, R. S., Lampert, J. & Sulo, S. (2012). Speaking up: Teens voice their health information needs. *Journal of School Nursing*, *28*(5), 379–388.

Spencer, G. (2013). Young people's perspectives on health: empowerment, or risk? *Health Education*, *113*(2), 115–131.

Stice, E., Marti, C. N., Shaw, H., & Jaconis, M. (2009). An 8-year longitudinal study of the natural history of threshold, subthreshold, and partial eating disorders from a community sample of adolescents. *Journal of Abnormal Psychology*, *118*, 587–597.

Suisman, J. L., O'Connor, S. M., Sperry, S., Thompson, J. K., Keel, P. K., Burt, S. A. ... Klump, K. L. (2012). Genetic and environmental influences on thin-ideal internalization. *International Journal of Eating Disorders*, *45*(8), 942–948.

Vacca, R., Vacca, J. & Begoray, D. (2005). *Content area reading: Literacy and learning across the curriculum*. Toronto, ON: Pearson Education.

Vardavas, C. I., Kondilis, B. K., Patelarou, E., Akrivos, P. D. & Falagas, M. E. (2009). Health literacy and sources of health education among adolescents in Greece. *International Journal of Adolescent Medicine & Health*, *21*(2), 179–186.

Wang, M.-T., Brinkworth, M. & Eccles, J. (2013). Moderating effects of teacher–student relationship in adolescent trajectories of emotional and behavioral adjustment. *Developmental Psychology*, *49*(4), 690–705.

West, A. E., Williams, E., Suzukovich, E., Strangeman, K. & Novins, D. (2012). A mental health needs assessment of urban American Indian youth and families. *American Journal of Community Psychology*, *49*(3–4), 441–453.

World Health Organization. (2014). *International day of the girl child*. Geneva, Switzerland: Author. Retrieved from http://www.who.int/ maternal_child_adolescent/news_events/ events/2014/girl-child-2014/en/

Zimmerman, M. A. (2013). Resiliency theory: A strengths-based approach to research and practice for adolescent health. *Health Education & Behavior*, *40*(4), 381–383.

In: Adolescent Health Literacy and Learning
Editors: D. L. Begoray and E. M. Banister

ISBN: 978-1-63482-897-0

Chapter 10

Looking Back and Looking Ahead

***Elizabeth Banister*[1,*] *and Deborah Begoray*[2]**
[1]School of Nursing, University of Victoria, Canada
[2]Department of Curriculum and Instruction, University of Victoria, Canada

Abstract

In this chapter, we discuss 3 main themes that provide an overview of adolescent health literacy and learning approaches as outlined by the authors in the preceding chapters. These themes are nurturing inquiry, engaging youth, and using bridging activities. We end with a discussion of 5 future trends, taking into consideration the complexity of adolescent worlds and the need for health educators and health systems to work harder to address adolescents as individuals and as a specific life-stage group. These trends are consideration of adolescent demography, growth of the importance of media and information technology, development of more relevant and responsive health education, adopting community-based approaches, and the creation of health-literate systems and institutions.

Keywords: critical inquiry, engaging youth, bridging activities, future trends

Introduction

Focusing Questions

1. What has emerged from this book as important to adolescent health literacy and learning?
2. How do health educators need to approach adolescents given the web of societal, cultural, community, family, and peer influences that impact their health behaviour patterns?

---

* Correspondence author: ebaniste@uvic.ca.

Adolescent Health Literacy and Learning describes the present but also looks to the future. Greater attention to adolescent health literacy is needed, given that adolescence is a "gateway" (Raphael, 2013, p. 137) period in an adolescent's life for enhancing health in the present and in their future adulthood. Authors in this book discuss a wide range of health topics and learning approaches used for enhancing adolescents' health literacy that will, in turn, build their capacity to make proactive health decisions and, thus, help them to attain better health (Ormshaw, Paakkari, & Kannas, 2013).

As editors of this book, we acknowledge the impact of a social ecology of individuals and groups on adolescents' health, in particular, that this population is situated in a dynamic web of societal, cultural, community, family, and peer influences that affect present and future health behaviour patterns and wellbeing (Viner et al., 2012). We encourage the development of an adolescent's critical thinking, sense of individual identity, social responsibility, and even social activism as part of their health literacy. In addition, we recognize the need for adolescents to have the "motivation, confidence, [and] trust" (Greenhalgh, 2015, p. 1) to put their knowledge into action. Thus, adolescent health literacy, like health literacy in other life stages, is multifaceted. It cannot be improved without both formal and informal learning opportunities for adolescents to engage with health knowledge, and an environment with knowledgeable adults who encourage and support such learning. The many contributors to *Adolescent Health Literacy and Learning* share these beliefs.

THEMES

Three common themes emerged from the chapters as important elements in adolescent health literacy and learning. These themes are nurturing inquiry, engaging youth, and using bridging activities.

Nurturing Inquiry

Nurturing an inquiring mind in adolescents is fundamental for their ability to think independently and make proactive health decisions. Health educators need to take into account the complexity of adolescent health and facilitate their ability to "think critically about the social, cultural, economic, political and environmental determinants of health and effect of these on themselves and on others" (Matthews, 2014, p. 2). Rather than *give* adolescents health information, which can undermine the development of independent thinking (Rogow, 2011), health educators need to *facilitate* adolescents' confidence in their own ability to reason; they need to nurture inquiry, open-mindedness, and consideration of alternative points of view (Facione, 1990). This nurturing includes creating learning environments that are supportive and non-threatening — that promote adolescents' ability to construct their own perspectives of health issues (Nutbeam, 2008) and to understand the perspectives of others (Paakkari & Paakkari, 2012).

Educators can engage learners in "critical enjoyment" (Redmond, 2012, p. 106) by creating learning environments that encourage co-learning, respect and inquiry that fosters "active and social learning in order to broaden students' experiences" (p. 113) in discussing health issues. In such environments, students learn to reflect on the relevance of health knowledge for their own lives and to proactively promote their own health and the health of others (Paakkari & Paakkari, 2012).

Adolescents need to be equipped to engage with and critically evaluate the credibility of health sources (Paakkari & Paakkari, 2012). This idea aligns with the concept of critical health literacy. Sykes, Wills, Rowlands, and Popple (2013) described evaluation as a higher order cognitive process that could be "developed through education to critically appraise information of relevance to health" (p. 2). Through reflection and dialogue, for example, adolescents learn to critique the underlying assumptions and values of health knowledge (Paakkari & Paakkari, 2012); they learn to find their own answers rather than have others impose these upon them (Matthews, 2014). To encourage this kind of critical analysis, educators need to use flexibility in the kinds of questions they pose that are contextually relevant to adolescents' learning situations and are developmentally appropriate (Rogow, 2011).

For example, Banister and Begoray, in chapter 5 (Teaching Middle Adolescents to Critically Reflect on the Interaction of Gender with Health Advertising) describe how an inquiry-based teaching practice that used critical questions in the research interview context encouraged middle school students to critically analyze media messages in terms of gender and health. It also involved them in reflection on the role of gender stereotyping in the health advertisements they created. As Redmond (2012) stated, this teaching practice "kindled students' satisfaction in the analytical, social, and expressive processes of media deconstruction" (p. 113) and provided space for them to develop an understanding of the media in their own terms. Critical analysis, active learning, and valuing of material selected by students encouraged learning at both the cognitive and affective levels (Redmond, 2012).

Incorporating a critical media health literacy framework, Begoray and Fu in chapter 3 (Reading *Chasing Adland*: Middle Years' Students in Pursuit of Critical Media Health Literacy) describe the use of dialogic inquiry (Reznitskaya, 2012). The teacher in this project engaged middle school students in raising questions about the characters, dialogue, and illustrations of a graphic novel about health advertising that had been created by another group of middle school students. The authors illustrated the value of inquiry in which both students and the classroom teacher were co-inquirers and collaboratively engaged in interpreting and evaluating the text.

In chapter 9 (Addressing Girls' Health Literacy and Learning with Young Adult 'Problem' Novels), Begoray, Banister, and Jaswal discuss the use of novels to promote adolescents to think critically about adverse health events (e.g., alcohol use, teen suicide, eating disorders, and bullying) they or their peers may encounter in the present or future. For example, in discussing the novel about a young Canadian Indigenous woman, *Tilly: A story of hope and resilience* (Gray Smith, 2013), the authors suggest that educators engage adolescents in critical conversations to make visible systems of oppression that Indigenous youth encounter on a daily basis.

Ranahan, in chapter 8 (Mental Health Literacies in Youth Work Practice with Adolescents), suggests that youth worker mental health literacy practice include the ability to critically examine structural factors that serve to oppress or limit supportive care. Critical reflection and questioning of structural systems and policies are fundamental to youth worker practice. Such mental health literacy can facilitate suicidal youth to proactively seek support and to engage in activities that are life sustaining.

Reporting on results from their study that examined students' responses to a high school health literacy curriculum in Yangon, Beer and Begoray in chapter 4 (High School Health Literacy in Burma/Myanmar) note that dialogue with peers about mental health through an online blog discussion forum, face-to-face discussions, and open-ended questions contributed to students' ability to ask questions and engage in dialogue about the credibility of health information. The authors found little evidence, however, of critical engagement within online social contexts (e.g., gaming communities).

Clearly, nurturing inquiry, especially through critical thinking, is a valuable approach to fostering adolescent health literacy and learning. To develop critical thinking skills, however, demands active participation of adolescents.

Engaging Youth

Adolescents' active engagement in identifying their health issues and developing solutions will help to raise the visibility of this population to their communities, to stakeholders, and to decision and policy makers (Sawyer et al., 2012). Learning is a process of social construction whereby knowledge is constructed by adolescent learners through interaction with others (Vygotsky, 1962); therefore, learning contexts need to be established in which students' background experiences and understanding of health are discussed collaboratively. Subject matters and materials need to be meaningful to the individual adolescents involved and also to their community. Rather than focus on narrow outcomes, health educators can establish learning contexts that encourage adolescents to connect them more broadly with health content, with their teachers and peers, and with the educational context and larger society (Redmond, 2012). For example, adolescents learn more effectively when they are actively engaged as co-learners in power-sharing situations that facilitate discussions inclusive of a range of perspectives and voices (Matthews, 2014).

In chapter 6 (Fast Food vs. Fitness: The Gendered Health Literacy Needs of High School Students), Wharf Higgins and Bellows Riecken discuss how engagement in a collective decision-making process for implementing school-based health information activities encouraged students to obtain and critically reflect on information relevant to their health. These discussions also offered students opportunities for engaging in health literacy practices outside of school.

Banister and Begoray, in chapter 5, describe middle school students' active participation in learning about media advertising in a classroom with peers and a teacher who valued their views (Redmond, 2012).

In chapter 7 (Integrating Culture to Enhance Mental Health Literacy among Aboriginal Youth), Marshall outlines how health educators can use a cultural approach to engage Aboriginal youth in their mental health literacy. These approaches might include youth-focused communication approaches such as validating nonverbal expressions and using a cultural consultant.

The importance of engaging adolescents in developing their health literacy is a theme taken up by several authors. Lifelong learning patterns can be established with adolescents taking active control of their health literacy development: accessing, understanding, evaluating, and communicating health information. Adult allies, however, often need to provide bridges to assist adolescents to reach this goal.

Using Bridging Activities

Adolescents need to be involved in health literacy in ways that are specific to their needs and interests. Authors in this book have considered what it might take to "bridge adolescents' everyday literacies with literacies common to subject areas" (Alvermann & Hinchman, 2012, p. 270). Health is an area of lifelong and life-wide importance to adolescents as they seek information and guidance for themselves and for their families, friends, and the wider communities in which they live. The bridging activities discussed in this book show that it is possible to place adolescents at centre stage and involve them in their health literacy.

Begoray and Fu, for example, in chapter 3 discuss a middle years classroom project that involved teens in creating a graphic novel and, subsequently, another group of adolescents in reading and discussing that same novel. Their teacher was excited to have an anchor text for use in health education and literacy education — a narrative they could return to as they continued to learn health literacy concepts. The students were keen to discuss the novel and to connect its ideas on critical thinking to their own lives and experiences with commercial media advertising.

In chapter 5, Banister and Begoray describe a multimedia project that involved middle school students in learning about media literacy and then creating their own video advertisements. These advertisements for healthy extracurricular activities were created for an authentic audience of their peers in their own school.

In chapter 8, Ranahan argues that new literacies are needed for effective practice with adolescents experiencing mental health issues that are absent in the current conceptualization. The author draws upon social learning theory and critical learning theory to offer a reconceptualization of mental health literacies that include relational knowledge or *being with* an adolescent who is contemplating suicide. Ranahan uses a case study to illustrate how a youth worker can approach a suicidal adolescent by communicating empathy, being fully present, and inviting a youth to share an experience. She suggests the use of a relational approach to facilitate adolescents' participation in identifying what help they need.

Throughout *Adolescent Health Literacy and Learning*, the three themes of nurturing inquiry, engaging youth, and using bridging activities appear and reappear in the work of our contributors. Defining and conceptualizing adolescent health literacy continues, however, to be a challenge, as Malloy-Weir discusses in chapter 2. This work will be needed in the future if this field of scholarship and research is to thrive. We see a number of other future trends as well in adolescent health literacy and learning.

Future Trends

Consideration of Adolescent Demography

Today's adolescents span two demographic groups. Older adolescents, the so-called Millennial generation, are heading into a world "more global and networked than in previous decades, … marked by increased knowledge and information transfer, heightened risks, fairly low social mobility, and greater economic inequality" (Institute of Medicine, 2014, p. 2). As a group, they tend to be distrustful of social institutions but optimistic about the future (Pew

Social Trends, 2014). We speculate that these trends may mean that health systems and schools will have to work harder to consider demographics to engage adolescents in ways they find appealing. In addition, we believe that trust and relationship building will be even more important than it is presently. Youth optimism about the future, however, works to our advantage in empowering them to build a better world.

Post Millennials, those born in 2000 or after, are growing up in a world characterized by turmoil caused by factors such as terrorism, labour unrest, job insecurity, and financial volatility (Caumont, 2014). The natural environment is at greater and greater risk. These adolescents are more technologically connected and socially aware than previous generations, which may, ironically, cause them greater anxiety about negative social events. They may also face extended adolescence as economic challenges stand in the way of complete independence. They are, however, idealistic and involved in helping to solve problems in new ways made possible by technology.

Growth of the Importance of Media and Information Technology

Over the past 40 years, adolescents have been exposed to a substantial increase in media and information technology (Viner et al., 2012) that they use, in part, as a way to establish independence from adult surveillance as they mature and, in part, to achieve and maintain connections with social networks. Rideout, Foehr, and Roberts (2010) estimated that total media time amongst 8- to 18-year-olds has risen to almost 11 hours per day — more than any other activity, including sleeping. Media sources can help to promote adolescent health; conversely, exposure to some content (e.g., cigarette and alcohol advertising) can negatively influence their health risk behaviours. Likewise, even though social media can offer opportunities for peer engagement, adolescents are vulnerable to the influence of intense exposure (e.g., reduced physical activities) and exposure to health-risk situations (e.g., cyberbullying or sexting, the transmission of sexually explicit messages) (Sawyer et al., 2010).

The saturation of media into adolescents' lives suggests the need for health educators to reduce its potential health risks and foster its appropriate use (Strasburger et al., 2013). It behooves us, therefore, to make health information readily available to adolescents using appropriate social media platforms. Second, we know that adolescents often turn to the Internet for information about sensitive health issues such as pregnancy and sexually transmitted infections. We need to equip adolescents to evaluate the quality of the significant amount of online information available to them. Educators and parents can, for example, inform adolescents of responsible health information sites such as *Go ask Alice* (http://goaskalice.columbia.edu), a health question-and-answer Internet resource for teens. Third, we need to assist adolescents to communicate accurate health information to their peers through face-to-face and technologically mediated approaches. Finally, we need to address health education in the schools to make it more nimble in the face of a barrage of information from other sources. We see the growth of media and technology influence on adolescent health literacy continuing and advancing in the future, likely on an even steeper trajectory.

Development of More Relevant and Responsive Health Education

We predict that schools will gradually change their approaches to meet adolescents' ways of learning. For example, the British Columbia (BC) Ministry of Education (2015) has adopted a personalized learning approach to education "where students have more opportunity to pursue their passions and interests" (p. 1). Students will have the chance in every subject to learn the basics but also to investigate topics of their own choosing, including, no doubt, questions surrounding health and wellness. Ontario has just introduced a new Health and Physical Education curriculum (Ontario Ministry of Education, 2015) that specifically names, defines, and integrates health literacy and tackles challenging topics such as sexual education. In addition, this curriculum specifies the importance of community partners such as public health units for achieving its goals. We see in the future that health literacy will be more specifically integrated into school curricula with a more defined role for the wider community in the education of individual students.

Adoption of Community-based Approaches

We know that many adolescents in developing countries worldwide but also in some communities in wealthy countries lack the health literacy to empower themselves to take more control over their health. There is, however, a trend to implement more community-based, participatory programs, such as Ontario's health curriculum discussed above and Australia's *OPHELIA* (*OP*timising *HE*alth *LI*teracy and *A*ccess to health information and services; Batterham et al., 2014). This program's authors offer health literacy learning approaches that include ways to adapt the curriculum to local cultural understandings about health; it is flexible and can be implemented with changes to create more relevant health reforms. *OPHELIA* was especially designed for reducing health inequalities in the general population. We anticipate that adolescents within these communities might be included as a subculture in need of further specific modifications. We know that the interaction of individuals and communities with health systems and institutions constitutes better overall health literacy improvement.

Creation of Health-literate Systems and Institutions

"[Health literacy] does not refer only to the ability and responsibility of individuals ... to become more health literate but also to the ability and responsibility of systems through which information relevant to health is provided" (Gillis, Begoray, & Rowlands, 2012, p. 2). If the interactions of adolescents with health practitioners are to be successful, each side must endeavour to work with the other. As adults, however, the onus lies on us to adjust health messaging, for example, to meet adolescent needs and work to reform systems that address adolescent health needs. Indeed, as Ranahan points out in chapter 8, adult allies must be prepared to challenge the system, including authority figures in health institutions, if allies are to effectively advocate for adolescents. We predict that this trend may be slow in developing and will need the ongoing attention of health literacy promoters if systems and institutional practices are to be modified for the benefit of adolescents.

As we decided on the trends in *Adolescent Health Literacy and Learning*, we became aware that there was more than a little wishful thinking in our prognostications. Nevertheless, our consideration of the work of adolescent health literacy scholars such as those represented in this book caused us to see the possibility of a more robust response to the needs of adolescents in the future and to be more convinced that these trends were likely.

CONCLUSION

We began this book by asserting that adolescent health was at a crucial juncture, but that adolescent health literacy and learning was understudied by researchers and underemphasized in the schools and other sites of health education. The many contributors to this book, however, offer tangible proof that there are positive steps being taken. Their work serves to offer hope to the field and models for others to follow. As we continue our work with adolescents, we welcome others to join and take up this most worthy cause. The health of our society in the future may well depend on how well we work with and for adolescents in the present!

Questions for Discussion, Reflection, and Writing

1. After reading this volume, what do you see as other themes arising from the contributors' discussions of adolescent health literacy and learning?
2. Why is it important that we consider future trends in adolescent health literacy and learning?

List of Online Resources

- Pew Research Center: Teens fact sheet – http://www.pewinternet.org/ fact-sheets/teens-fact-sheet/
- Common Sense Education: Helping Teens Find Health Information Online They Can Trust – https://www.commonsensemedia.org/ educators/blog/helping-teens-find-health-information-online-they-can-trust

REFERENCES

Alvermann, D. E. & Hinchman, K. A. (2012). Afterword. In D. E. Alvermann & K. A. Hinchman (Eds.), *Reconceptualizing the literacies in adolescents' lives: Bridging the everyday/academic divide* (3rd ed., 270–274). New York, NY: Routledge.

Batterham, R. W., Buchbinder, R., Beauchamp, A., Dodson, S., Elsworth, G. T. & Osborne, R. H. (2014). The OPtimising HEalth LIterAcy (OPHELIA) process: Study protocol for using health literacy profiling and community engagement to create and implement health reform. *BMC Public Health*, *14*, 694. doi:10.1186/1471-2458-14-694

British Columbia Ministry of Education. (2015). *BC's education plan: Focus on learning.* Victoria, BC: Author. Retrieved from http://www. bcedplan.ca/assets/pdf/bcs_education_plan_2015.pdf

Caumont, A. (2014, March 12). *What would you name today's youngest generation of Americans?* (Factank: News in the Numbers). Washington, DC: Pew Research Center. Retrieved from http://www.pewresearch.org/ fact-tank/2014/03/12/what-would-you-name-todays-youngest-generation-of-americans/

Facione, P. A. (1990). *Critical thinking: A statement of expert consensus for purposes of educational assessment and instruction* (Executive Summary). Millbrae, CA: California Academic Press. Retrieved from http://assessment.aas.duke.edu/documents/Delphi_Report.pdf

Gillis, D., Begoray, D. & Rowlands, G. (2012). Introducing health literacy in context. In D. Begoray, D. Gillis & G. Rowlands (Eds.), *Health literacy in context: International perspectives* (1-12). Hauppage, NY: Nova Science.

Gray Smith, M. (2013). *Tilly: A story of hope and resilience.* Winlaw, BC: Sono Nis Press.

Greenhalgh, T. (2015). Health literacy: Towards system level solutions. *British Medical Journal, 350*, h1026, 1–2.

Institute of Medicine. (2014). *Investing in the health and well-being of young adults.* Washington, DC: National Academies Press. Retrieved from http://www.nap.edu/catalog/18869/investing-in-the-health-and-well-being-of-young-adults

Matthews, C. (2014). Critical pedagogy in health education. *Health Education Journal, 73*(5), 600–609.

Nutbeam, D. (2008). The evolving concept of health literacy. *Social Science and Medicine, 67*(1), 2072–2078.

Ontario Ministry of Education. (2015). *Health and physical education curriculum.* Toronto, ON: Queen's Printer for Ontario. Retrieved from http://www.edu.gov.on.ca/eng/curriculum/elementary/health1to8.pdf

Ormshaw, M. J., Paakkari, L. & Kannas, L. K. (2013). Measuring child and adolescent health literacy: A systematic review of literature. *Health Education, 113*(5), 433–455.

Paakkari, L. & Paakkari, O. (2012). Health literacy as a learning outcome in schools. *Health Education, 112*(2), 133–152.

Pew Social Trends. (2014, March 7). *Millennials in adulthood.* Washington, DC: Pew Research Center. Retrieved from http://www. pewsocialtrends.org/2014/03/07/millennials-in-adulthood/

Raphael, D. (2013). Adolescence as a gateway to adult health outcomes. *Maturitas, 75*(2), 137–141.

Redmond, T. (2012). The pedagogy of critical enjoyment: Teaching and reaching the hearts and minds of adolescent learners through media literacy education. *Journal of Media Literacy Education, 4*(2), 106–120.

Reznitskaya, A. (2012). Dialogic teaching: Rethinking language use during literature discussions. *The Reading Teacher, 65*(7), 446–456.

Rideout, V. J., Foehr, U. G. & Roberts, D. F. (2010). *Generation M^2: Media in the lives of 8- to 18-year-olds.* Menlo Park, CA: Henry J. Kaiser Family Foundation. Retrieved from https://kaiserfamilyfoundation. files.wordpress.com/2013/04/8010.pdf

Rogow, F. (2011). Ask, don't tell: Pedagogy for media literacy education in the next decade. *Journal of Media Literacy Education, 3*(1), 16–22.

Sawyer, S. M., Afifi, R. A., Bearinger, L. H., Blakemore, S. J., Dick, B., Ezeh, A. C. & Patton, G. C. (2012). Adolescence: A foundation for future health. *The Lancet*, *379*(9826), 1630–1640.

Strasburger, V. C., Hogan, M. J., Mulligan, D. A., Ameenuddin, N., Christakis, D. A., Cross, C. ... Swanson, W. S. L. (2013). Children, adolescents, and the media. *Pediatrics*, *132*(5), 958–961.

Sykes, S., Wills, J., Rowlands, G. & Popple, K. (2013). Understanding critical health literacy: A concept analysis. *BMC Public Health*, *13*(Feb.), Art. 150. doi:10.1186/1471-2458-13-150.

Viner, R. M., Ozer, E. M., Denny, S., Marmot, M., Resnick, M., Fatusi, A. & Currie, C. (2012). Adolescence and the social determinants of health. *The Lancet*, *379*(9826), 1641–1652.

Vygotsky, L. S. (1962). *Thought and language*. Cambridge, MA: MIT Press.

INDEX

A

B

C

D

E

F

G

H

I

K

L

M